AUSTSWIM

Australian Council for the Teaching of Swimming and Water Safety

2ND EDITION

AUSTSWIM

Australian Council for the Teaching of Swimming and Water Safety

2ND EDITION

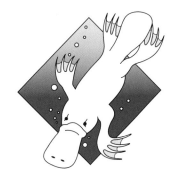

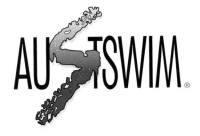

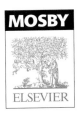

MOSBY

ELSEVIER

Sydney   Edinburgh   London   New York   Philadelphia   St Louis   Toronto

ELSEVIER

Mosby
is an imprint of Elsevier

Elsevier Australia
(a division of Reed International Books Australia Pty Ltd)
Tower 1, 475 Victoria Avenue, Chatswood, NSW 2067
ACN 001 002 357

Second edition © 2008 AUSTSWIM Limited; photos and illustrations © Elsevier Australia
Reprinted 2009, 2010, 2011, 2012
First edition © 2002 AUSTSWIM Limited

National Library of Australia Cataloguing-in-Publication Data

Teaching swimming and water safety : the Australian way.

2nd ed.
ISBN 978 1 875897 87 2 (pbk.).

1. Swimming - Study and teaching - Australia. 2. Aquatic
sports - Safety measures - Study and teaching - Australia.
I. Austswim.

797.21071094

Publishing Manager: Melinda McEvoy
Publishing Services Manager: Helena Klijn
Editorial Coordinator: Lauren Allsop
Edited and indexed by Forsyth Publishing Services
Proofread by Pamela Dunne
Illustrations by Greg Gaul
Photography by Harvie Allison
Cover and internal design by Jennifer Pace
Typeset by Sunset Digital Pty Ltd
Printed in China by China Translation and Printing Services

Where possible, Elsevier Australia endeavours to print on paper manufactured from sustainable forests.

CONTENTS

Chapter 10 Plan, deliver and review a lesson

Appendices

FOREWORD

AUSTSWIM has gained an outstanding national and international reputation for the training of quality teachers of swimming and water safety. Government, the aquatic industry and the community recognise AUSTSWIM awards as the industry standard for teachers of swimming and water safety.

The high-quality courses from AUSTSWIM have been enhanced by manuals and associated learning materials which cater for the teacher-training needs of a rapidly expanding and vibrant aquatic industry.

This manual represents the next step in AUSTSWIM's commitment to continuous improvement and quality outcomes and as such represents a significant step forward in providing an enhanced experience for students. The improved design and presentation will further assist course candidates to acquire the appropriate knowledge and skills to become competent teachers in aquatic education.

The topics deemed necessary for learning all aspects of teaching swimming and water safety are covered by this manual. While these skills are being developed, every opportunity is taken to impart water safety knowledge, to reduce the likelihood of aquatic incidents, including drownings.

Other AUSTSWIM publications cover the specialist areas of teaching swimming and water safety to infants, adults and people with a disability, and competitive strokes.

This manual plays a pivotal role in facilitating the delivery of quality swimming and water safety programs throughout Australia.

Kirk Marks
Chairman
AUSTSWIM Limited
2008

Gordon Mallett
Chief Executive Officer
AUSTSWIM Limited
2008

ACKNOWLEDGMENTS

AUSTSWIM gratefully acknowledges the contributions made to this manual and previous editions by AUSTSWIM staff, member organisations and individuals.

AUSTSWIM also acknowledges the following individuals and organisations for their contributions to this manual:

- Peter Conochie, Warren Curnow, Karen Franceschini, Meredith King, Penny Larsen, Susan Sturt and Ted Tullberg
- Lander and Rogers Lawyers — 'Legal responsibilities for the AUSTSWIM teacher', Chapter 2
- Royal Life Saving Society Australia (RLSSA) — 'Aquatic safety, survival and rescue skills', Chapter 5
- Melissa van Poppel — 'Principles of movement in water', Chapter 6
- Jenny Blitvich PhD, University of Ballarat — 'Teaching safer diving skills', Chapter 8
- Kirk Marks — 'Towards efficient stroke development', Chapter 9
- Dr George Janko, Sport & Spinal Physician, Medical Director McKinnon Sports Medicine — 'Medical considerations', Appendix 4.

AUSTSWIM gratefully acknowledges the ongoing contribution of RLSSA to this manual and other AUSTSWIM publications. People wishing to pursue other educational programs in water safety, swimming, survival, lifeguarding and resuscitation are encouraged to contact RLSSA at www.rlssa.org.au.

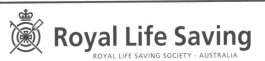

AUSTSWIM would also like to acknowledge the ongoing contribution of Surf Life Saving Australia (SLSA) to the AUSTSWIM publications. People wishing to find out more about SLSA awards, programs and services are encouraged to contact SLSA at www.slsa.asn.au.

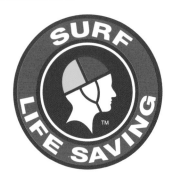

Whatever it takes.

AUSTSWIM also acknowledges the role of Swimming Australia Ltd (SAL) for its ongoing contribution to AUSTSWIM resource development. For further information about programs and services offered contact SAL at www.swimming.org.au.

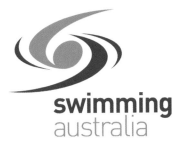

AUSTSWIM also wishes to acknowledge the generous support provided by the Commonwealth Government, through the Department of Health and Ageing.

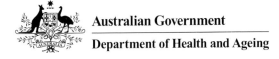

Overview of AUSTSWIM and the aquatic industry

CHAPTER 1

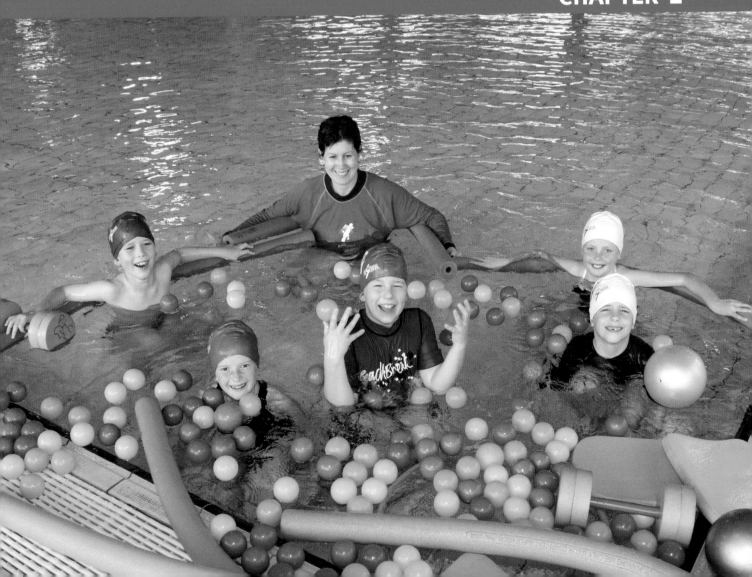

THE HISTORY OF AUSTSWIM

During the 1960s Australia experienced considerable changes, evidenced by improved affluence and an increased amount of leisure time. Participation in aquatic recreational pursuits increased significantly and home swimming pools were built at an ever-increasing rate.

Associated with this increase was the corresponding number of aquatic accidents and injuries. One significant reaction to this was to question the content of traditional swimming and water safety programs.

The commercial sector perceived the need to improve instructional programs, and many heated swimming pools were built with the major objective of providing first-class, year-round swimming tuition for all age groups. The success of the commercial swimming sector prompted local governments to re-evaluate their provision of leisure services; consequently, many councils built heated pools to cater for the year-round aquatic recreational needs of the community.

With facilities available for year-round swimming, traditional instruction methods came under increased scrutiny. Departments of education began to offer swimming and water safety programs to children from the lower years in primary school rather than to upper-year pupils; this enhanced the prospect of pupils becoming competent swimmers and possessing the desired survival and safety skills prior to leaving primary school.

During this period of change a number of concerns were expressed in regard to learn-to-swim programs. They included:

- a lack of unity in relation to acceptable qualifications and the degree of experience of swimming teachers
- a disparity of opinion regarding methods of teaching swimming, survival and rescue techniques to various age and ability groups
- the proliferation of certificates and awards available to participants with no quality assurance methods in place
- a range of standards demonstrated by candidates in obtaining certificates and awards.

A national forum was conducted in Melbourne during 1979 with the view of establishing a national organisation responsible for the teaching of swimming and water safety. Delegates at the forum voted unanimously in favour of this, and the Australian Council for the Teaching of Swimming and Water Safety (AUSTSWIM) was formed with the major objective of developing a sound educational base for this teaching.

The structure of AUSTSWIM

AUSTSWIM is Australia's leading organisation for the training of teachers of swimming and water safety. AUSTSWIM is a not-for-profit organisation that has a business centre or equivalent in each state and territory of Australia. The AUSTSWIM Council comprises an independent chairperson, a representative from each state and territory and a representative from six major aquatic organisations — Swimming Australia Ltd, the Royal Life Saving Society Australia, Surf Life Saving Australia, YMCA Australia, the Australian Leisure Facilities Association and Water Safety New Zealand.

AUSTSWIM has recently undergone a restructure that has seen the organisation move from having a traditional federation structure to a streamlined corporate model. A federation model is best described as one which has a number of independent state and territory organisations reporting to a national organisation, which is how most national sporting organisations are structured.

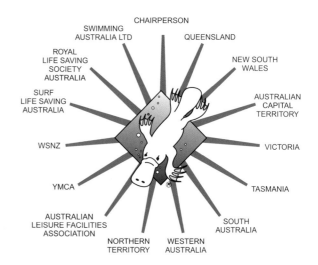

The AUSTSWIM Council

AUSTSWIM'S VISION

AUSTSWIM's vision is that every Australian will be taught to swim by an accredited AUSTSWIM teacher, enabling them to safely enjoy aquatic environments and activities.

AUSTSWIM'S MISSION

- AUSTSWIM Leadership
- AUSTSWIM Standards
- AUSTSWIM Products and Services
- AUSTSWIM Licensing

AUSTSWIM'S VALUES

At AUSTSWIM we strive to:

- demonstrate the highest ethical and professional standards in our dealings with customers
- create an environment which promotes the value of learning and education
- acknowledge our staff as a fundamental and an important resource necessary to the sustainability of the organisation
- provide and add value to our customers through their learning
- nurture a culture of being approachable, informal, supportive, flexible and open
- be mindful of our history and build on past experience and the philosophies of AUSTSWIM
- provide equity of access to the delivery of our service.

Relationship with member organisations

AUSTSWIM has a close philosophical and working relationship with the following organisations. The national meetings of AUSTSWIM provide an excellent forum for them to share knowledge and to discuss issues of common interest. A spirit of cooperation exists between the organisations, with the health and welfare of all Australians being of prime consideration.

SWIMMING AUSTRALIA LTD (SAL)

Swimming Australia Ltd (SAL) is the peak body for competitive swimming in Australia. There are nine stakeholders consisting of seven state and territory swimming associations, the Australian Swimmers' Association (ASA) and the Australian Swimming Coaches and Teachers Association Inc (ASCTA). SAL currently has approximately 100,000 registered members in over 900 swimming clubs nationally. The members include swimmers, officials, administrators, coaches and volunteers. SAL is responsible for the management and development of the sport from the 'grass-roots' participation level through to the national team at elite level.

SAL is the body responsible for the accreditation of all swimming coaches through the National Coaches Accreditation Scheme (NCAS). SAL recognises the AUSTSWIM qualification as the primary accreditation for learn-to-swim teachers and recognises the skills that such teachers bring if they wish to progress on to coaching. Swimming teachers are encouraged to advance their skills in the development of the swimming strokes and swimming coaching techniques through the Green, Bronze, Silver and Gold Licence coaching accreditation courses provided. Like AUSTSWIM, there is a vocational outcome available for accredited swimming coaches of club swimmers within the SAL structure.

SAL provides the structure that supports competitive swimming opportunities for all ages and all abilities with club, interclub, regional, state, territory, national and international level meets.

SAL works closely with ASCTA to provide professional development opportunities for coaches throughout Australia.

For more information go to:
www.swimming.org.au

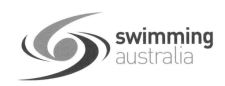

THE ROYAL LIFE SAVING SOCIETY AUSTRALIA (RLSSA)

The Royal Life Saving Society Australia (RLSSA) is the leading water safety, swimming and lifesaving education organisation in Australia. The RLSSA is a nationwide organisation that has been educating millions of Australians for over 100 years.

The mission of the RLSSA is 'To prevent loss of life and injury in the community with an emphasis on aquatic environments'. The RLSSA pursues this mission through:

- water safety programs
- lifesaving training programs
- aquatic safety audits and risk management services
- advocacy and public awareness
- lifesaving sporting opportunities.

The four main RLSSA water safety programs that AUSTSWIM teachers may be involved in are:

1. Infant Aquatics — the program's key components are water familiarisation, water safety and early stroke development with a focus on learning and experiencing a range of skills in a fun, safe and non-threatening environment.
2. Swim and Survive — a program aimed towards 5 to 14 year olds developing swimming technique, water safety knowledge, water confidence, survival skills and endurance integrated through a range of aquatic skills.
3. Bronze Rescue — focuses on developing survival and rescue skills with the ability to make safe judgments that may help individuals or others survive an aquatic emergency.
4. Junior Lifeguard Club — a unique alternative aquatic program for those who wish to further develop aquatic skills and lifesaving knowledge.

The RLSSA has a range of educational resources to support each of the water safety programs to assist teachers in delivering quality swimming, water safety and lifesaving lessons.

For more information go to:

www.royallifesaving.com.au.

EVERYONE CAN BE A LIFESAVER

Royal Life Saving
ROYAL LIFE SAVING SOCIETY - AUSTRALIA

SURF LIFE SAVING AUSTRALIA (SLSA)

Surf Life Saving Australia (SLSA) is the largest volunteer water safety and rescue organisation in the world. Over 300 of Australia's beaches are patrolled by 25,000 active surf lifesavers representing 303 surf lifesaving clubs in every state and in the Northern Territory.

The aims of SLSA are:

- to supply services that minimise danger and prevent loss of life or injury in beach and other aquatic environments
- to educate the community in beach and aquatic safety and to promote skills and knowledge in beach and surf recreation
- to gain recognition in the community as the authority and provider of information on matters related to beach and aquatic safety and management.

SLSA provides an extensive safety network according to community needs; this incorporates comprehensive motorised craft, rescue helicopters, radio networks, advanced resuscitation equipment, community displays, seminars and promotions of beach and aquatic safety messages, special-event water safety services and the Australian Beach Safety and Management Program. SLSA (through its subsidiary Australian Lifeguard Services) is also the largest employer of professional lifeguards in the country, who patrol beaches around Australia on either a full- or a part-time basis.

For more information go to:

www.slsa.com.au

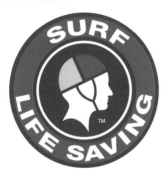

Whatever it takes.

YMCA AUSTRALIA

The YMCA is a community-based charity helping to build strong people, families and communities.

In partnership with government, non-profit groups and associates, over 500,000 Australians participate in the Y's seven core areas of:

- accommodation
- aquatics
- camping and outdoor education
- children's services
- health and wellbeing
- sport and recreation
- youth services.

YMCA Australia's commitment to swimming and water safety delivers community education through the AquaSafe Aquatic Education Program.

AquaSafe

AquaSafe presents a unique opportunity to develop skills and share experiences in an aquatic environment. The program promotes confidence, self awareness and social interaction combined with swimming and water safety knowledge and skills.

AquaSafe infant and preschool program

Parental education is a major focus—children are joined in class to support the learning process, enhance water safety elements and foster safe aquatic practices. Learning outcomes in infant classes include:

- water safety
- body orientation and coordination skills
- introduction to floating, propulsion, entry and exit.

AquaSafe primary program

Progressive modules challenge students to develop increasing endurance, strive for improvement, think for themselves and respect the aquatic environment.

Learning outcomes in primary classes focus on three distinctive areas:

Intellectual development:

- Decision making
- Problem solving
- Self confidence
- Teamwork

Physical development:

- Water safety
- Stroke development
- Exercise
- Coordination

Personal development:

- Talking
- Listening
- Cooperation
- Respect

YMCA and AUSTSWIM

YMCA Australia supports AUSTSWIM and is a large employer of AUSTSWIM Teachers of Swimming and Water Safety. For more information go to www.ymca.org.au.

We build strong **PEOPLE**
strong **FAMILIES** strong **COMMUNITIES**

AUSTRALIAN LEISURE FACILITIES ASSOCIATION (ALFA)

The Australian Leisure Facilities Association (ALFA) is the peak representative body for the aquatic, recreation and leisure facilities industry in Australia. Although only established in 2009, ALFA has a pedigree with aquatics and facilities dating back over 75 years, and was formed out of a strong industry need for a national organisation to represent its interests.

Facilities are at the heart of aquatics, recreation and leisure provision and are essential to the continuing development of a healthy Australian community. ALFA's vision is to 'Raise the quality, increase usage and improve the customer experience relating to aquatic, recreation and leisure facilities in Australia'.

To achieve this vision ALFA focuses on advocacy for key industry issues, providing leadership on industry policies and standards, ensuring relevant professional development opportunities, and sharing latest industry trends and knowledge through strong networks and membership communications. ALFA represents individual employees, organisations that own, manage or lease facilities, and companies that supply to the industry, offering Individual, Organisation and Commercial Supplier memberships.

ALFA is the national voice for the industry, and has strong local networks. Members of ALFA are also members of the ALFA recognised industry body in their state or territory. For more information go to www.alfaleisure.org.au.

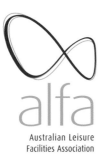

alfa
Australian Leisure
Facilities Association

WATER SAFETY NEW ZEALAND

Formed in 1949 Water Safety New Zealand (WSNZ) is the national organisation responsible for water safety education in New Zealand. WSNZ is a membership based collective comprising 36 member organisations that elect the Board that governs the national office. WSNZ is the collective organisation responsible for ensuring that all New Zealanders are educated to be safe in, on and around the water. WSNZ provides leadership in water safety education and the prevention of drowning.

Our Vision

Everyone in New Zealand will have the water safe skills and behaviours necessary to use and enjoy the water safely.

Our Mission

Through water safety education, prevent injury and drowning

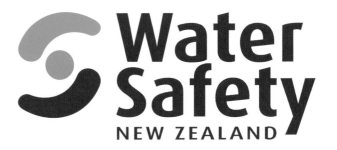

Water
Safety
NEW ZEALAND

AUSTSWIM'S TRAINING PROGRAM

AUSTSWIM has developed a quality training program for those wishing to enter the aquatic industry as a teacher of swimming and water safety. AUSTSWIM registration is the minimum industry standard for swimming and water safety teachers.

AUSTSWIM teachers are eligible to instruct a variety of age and ability groups, appropriate to the current certificate held, including:

- infants and preschoolers
- school-aged children
- adults
- people with a disability.

Participants who successfully complete course requirements for an AUSTSWIM training program are registered for a period of 3 years. After this time AUSTSWIM teachers are required to re-register with AUSTSWIM.

The AUSTSWIM training program is delivered and recognised in each state and territory of Australia, and many countries overseas, and can lead to other career opportunities within the industry. As the entry point qualification into aquatic teaching, the AUSTSWIM teacher may choose to also gain additional qualifications or further their career pathways in the industry into areas such as coordinating aquatic programs, lifeguarding, swim coaching and facility management.

AUSTSWIM TEACHER OF SWIMMING AND WATER SAFETY

Candidates may enrol into an extension course but cannot receive the extension teacher licence until the AUSTSWIM Teacher of Swimming and Water Safety Teacher Licence is completed.

EXTENSION COURSES
- AUSTSWIM Teacher of Infant and Preschool Aquatics
- AUSTSWIM Teacher of Aquatics for People with a Disability
- AUSTSWIM Teacher of Towards Competitive Strokes
- AUSTSWIM Teacher of Adults

REVIEW QUESTIONS

1 What is AUSTSWIM's vision?
2 List the AUSTSWIM elective courses available.
3 Once qualified, how often is an AUSTSWIM teacher required to re-register with AUSTSWIM?
4 Who are the member organisations of AUSTSWIM?

Legal responsibilities for the AUSTSWIM teacher

CHAPTER 2

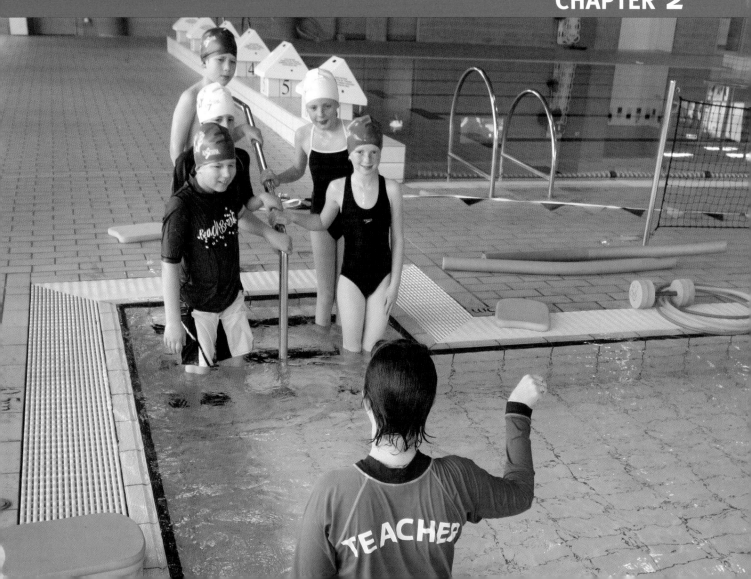

LEGAL LIABILITY

The law imposes standards of behaviour on us all. Being in a position of authority and responsibility, the swimming and water safety teacher should be clearly aware of what the law expects of them, for it is clear that swimming and water safety teachers are not immune from legal liability.

The purpose of this chapter is to outline the various areas of legal liability that a swimming and water safety teacher may be subject to. It highlights the need for swimming and water safety teachers to adopt a risk management strategy to minimise the risks arising in the first place. When working in and around water, there is a certain degree of risk. Swimming and water safety teachers must behave in a reasonable manner to ensure that the people they are teaching are not subjected to unreasonable risk or harm. Preventing the risk arising in the first place is the best way of limiting legal liability.

There are essentially four areas of the law that swimming and water safety teachers need to be aware of:

1. negligence
2. contract law
3. criminal law
4. harassment/discrimination.

In addition, swimming and water safety teachers should be familiar with the following legal concepts and principles:

1. privacy
2. risk management
3. insurance
4. natural justice.

BE AWARE AND PREPARE
- Do you hold a current AUSTSWIM registration?
- Do you hold a current CPR certificate?
- Do you have insurance cover?
- Know your duty of care.
- Adopt a risk management program.

Negligence

Negligence is the most common claim that a swimming and water safety teacher is likely to face.

If a court finds that a swimming and water safety teacher has acted negligently in the performance of their duty and someone has suffered loss or injury as a result, the court is likely to require the swimming and water safety teacher to compensate the injured person for their loss or injury. Depending on the circumstances, other parties such as the owner of the premises or the employer of the swimming and water safety teacher may also be liable to pay damages.

In order for a claim of negligence to be successful, four elements need to be established, namely that:

1. a duty of care was owed to the injured person
2. there was a breach of the duty of care
3. an injury or loss was suffered
4. there was a reasonable connection between the breach of duty of care and that injury or loss.

DUTY OF CARE

A duty of care in law is based on the concept of looking after your neighbour. In law, your neighbour is a person who is closely and directly affected by your actions. A duty of care will generally exist between a teacher and student given the close nature of the relationship between them. The duty imposed on the swimming and water safety teacher will depend on the circumstances, however it will entail the teacher avoiding causing or contributing to harm to another where that harm is foreseeable.

The law may also, depending on the circumstances, impose a duty of care on a swimming and water safety teacher for others in the vicinity, such as parents or other teachers. Again, the circumstances where this may occur will relate to whether the act or omissions of the teacher may cause or contribute to harm to those people.

BREACH OF THE DUTY OF CARE

Whether there has been a breach of the duty of care owed by a swimming and water safety teacher will be determined by the standard of care expected of the swimming and water safety teacher. The law will look at what a reasonable person would have done in the circumstances.

The courts will decide what is a reasonable standard of care by which a swimming and water safety teacher should be judged. Failure to adhere to the reasonable standard of care is likely to result in breach of the duty of care. Breach of the duty of care must be assessed on a case-by-case basis. There are no fixed rules to guide the behaviour of swimming and water safety teachers, but generally the courts will require that a swimming and water safety teacher behaves in a manner which is reasonable in the circumstances.

It follows that a duty may be imposed in situations outside set class times, and swimming and water safety teachers should consider what is reasonable in circumstances such as a parent running late to pick up a student, or the level of supervision prior to set class times. For example, it may be inappropriate to leave students alone to wait in an area which may be unsafe or dark, or to leave them at certain times of the day or night. In order to assess what is reasonable in the circumstances, swimming and water safety teachers should consider the factors noted below.

In determining the standard of care expected of a swimming and water safety teacher towards students, the following factors may be taken into account:

- the type of activity
- the characteristics of the student
- the swimming and water safety teacher's training and experience.

The type of activity

Generally, the more hazardous the activity, the greater the standard of care expected of a swimming and water safety teacher in relation to their student.

The range of water conditions and aquatic activities that may be encountered in a broad swimming program is considerable, and therefore the required level of care will be constantly changing. Even in the timeframe of one lesson, the standard of care can change simply by movement of the students from shallow to deep water.

Swimming and water safety teachers should be aware of this variation in the standard of care and increase their alertness and degree of supervision when required. It may be necessary to alter teaching techniques if the practising of a particular skill requires a lower swimming teacher–student ratio. The degree of danger inherent in a particular activity must determine the necessary standard of care.

Swimming and water safety teachers should also consider the hazards involved in activities outside class time, including periods prior to or after classes where young students may have to wait without supervision.

The characteristics of the student

Age

As a general rule, the younger the student, the higher the standard of care that is owed. For example, a young baby may not survive without adult assistance, whereas an independent, mature 15 year old who is competent would not require the same amount of supervision and assistance. However, a frail adult in a class for older people may require a higher standard of care than a fit and active, water-competent person of 55.

A duty of care still applies when the student is an adult. However, because the standard of care depends on the circumstances, it is likely to be lower than for the student who is a child.

Ability

Swimming and water safety teachers should not consider the age of the student in isolation. It is important to assess the student's ability before any tasks are allocated. While it is important to challenge and extend students in a swimming and water safety program, they must not be instructed to undertake activities that are beyond their capabilities nor be put in environments in which there is a likelihood of injury. Obviously beginners need greater supervision than more experienced and skilled students.

Physical capability

The standard of care will also vary according to the physical capability of the student. Swimming and water safety teachers must be acutely aware of each student's physical capabilities, taking appropriate precautions where necessary and providing supervision appropriate

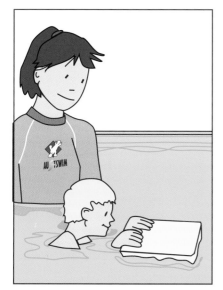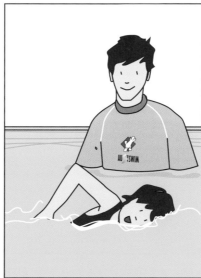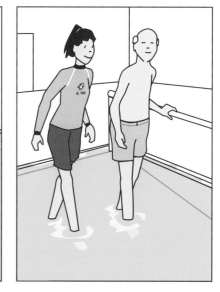

Your level of duty of care can alter depending on the age of the student

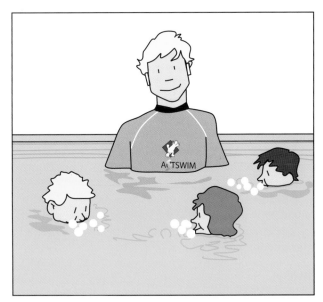
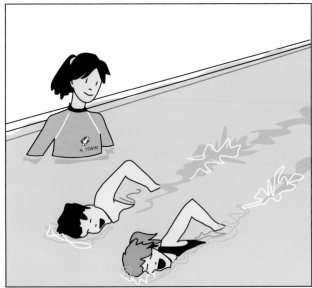

The ability of the student needs to be assessed prior to allocating tasks

for each one's needs. For example, a higher standard of care will be required when the student is an adult with a disability, as opposed to an adult without a disability.

Language and learning difficulties

Extra care must be taken to ensure that instructions are properly understood by students whose first language is not English, or by those who may have learning/comprehension difficulties, before they are permitted to attempt an activity.

Behaviour

If a student persistently disobeys the class or pool rules, steps must be taken to ensure that the behaviour does not result in an injury to themselves or others. A behaviour management plan should be part of every program. Emotionally disturbed children, or children with persistent behaviour problems may require additional supervision or behavioural management strategies.

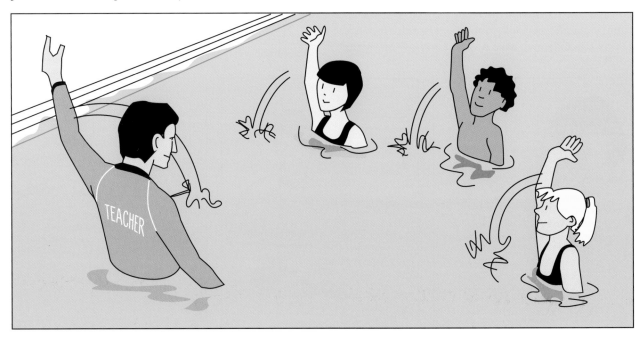

Extra care should be taken to ensure instructions are clear for students whose first language is not English

The swimming and water safety teacher's training and experience

The standard of care expected of a swimming and water safety teacher corresponds directly with the standard expected of a person possessing such qualifications. Therefore, AUSTSWIM teachers will be expected to make decisions using their training and experience. Thus, they have a higher standard of care imposed on them than a person without qualifications and experience.

INJURY SUSTAINED AND CONNECTION BETWEEN BREACH OF THE DUTY OF CARE AND THE INJURY SUSTAINED

For liability to be established, it must be shown that the student has suffered a loss or injury as a result of the breach of duty of care owed to them. Further, the loss or injury must not be too remote (that is, it must have been foreseeable that if the swimming and water safety teacher breached their duty, the student would be injured).

For example, an injury to a student due to a loose tile on the side of the pool may not be found to have been foreseeable if the poolside tiles had been recently installed, regularly maintained and no similar incidents had occurred. However, an identical incident may well be found to have been foreseeable if complaints had been received about the state of the tiling, and other students had experienced difficulty in relation to loose tiles prior to the injury occurring.

'COMMON PRACTICE'

A claim by a swimming and water safety teacher that they have acted in accordance with common practice is not necessarily a defence if the common practice is not considered to be reasonable. This is especially relevant to swimming and water safety teachers commencing a program at a particular venue. They should not rely on established procedures and continue to implement unsafe practices just because they have always been done that way.

For example, student–teacher ratios should not be accepted blindly, but must be considered in relation to the circumstances. If a class consists of very young children or the class is known to present behaviour problems, or if the swimming and water safety teacher is using natural water venues, the swimming student–teacher ratios may need to be adjusted in order to take into account all the particular risks inherent in that situation.

Summary

- Swimming and water safety teachers are unlikely to be found liable in a claim of negligence against them if they can show that they acted reasonably (i.e. as a reasonable person would have acted) in the circumstances.
- In maintaining the standard of care, swimming and water safety teachers should use ordinary commonsense together with experience and knowledge.
- The swimming and water safety teacher should attempt to use good judgment in all circumstances.
- The unplanned or hasty act is far more likely to involve risks which may result in a negligence claim than the well-planned action, even though the final result may be exactly the same.

Contract law

WHAT IS A CONTRACT?

A contract is a legally binding and enforceable agreement reached between two parties. A contract may be expressed in writing, orally, or implied by the conduct or actions of the parties.

A contract need not necessarily be in writing, although it is highly recommended that it is, so that the intentions of the contract are clear between the parties (and to any arbitrator called upon to resolve a dispute) from the outset.

For example, an oral statement by a pool owner that a swimming and water safety teacher is entitled to 15 per cent of all memberships signed up through his or her classes may constitute a legally binding contract regardless of the fact that the statement is not documented in a written contract.

A contract can be contrasted with a free promise, which is characterised by the lack of reward received by the party performing the task. A free promise is unenforceable unless it is contained in a deed which is a signed, sealed and delivered document. An example of a free promise might be where a parent volunteers to coach the junior squad each Sunday morning. If the parent reneges on this promise, they cannot be held to be in breach of contract.

CONTRACTS RELEVANT TO SWIMMING AND WATER SAFETY TEACHERS

Swimming and water safety teachers may enter into a whole host of contracts whether they realise it or not. These contracts may be formally documented or oral. Examples of such contracts include:

- employment contracts under which the swimming and water safety teacher is employed by a venue or organisation to coach or take swimming lessons
- sponsorship agreements where a local business may agree to provide money or donations to a junior team travelling interstate for a swim meet
- leasing premises such as a pool and change rooms for the conduct of swimming and water safety lessons
- purchasing equipment, which constitutes a contract between the seller of the equipment and the purchaser
- government funding often comes with contractual obligations on the recipient to use the funding in certain ways, behave in a proper fashion, or to submit to a drug-testing regime
- supply contracts for teaching services often have the same practical effect as an employment contract, however the relationship between the parties is one of independent contractor rather than employee/employer. The contract may be with a venue, or the individual student (or his or her parents)
- insurance contracts such as professional indemnity, or third party insurance.

ESSENTIAL ELEMENTS OF A CONTRACT

Essential elements to a legally binding contract are:

1 the **offer**, which requires a definite undertaking by the person making the offer to be bound if the offer is accepted
2 **acceptance**, which establishes the point in time the contract begins and which must be clear, certain and in response to the offer made
3 **consideration** (value attached to the agreement) such as the exchange of money, or a promise to do, or not to do something
4 an **intention to create legal relations** between the parties
5 **legal capacity** of parties — for instance, a contract is unlikely to be enforceable against a person who does not have legal capacity, such as a minor, an unincorporated association (which does not have a legal entity separate from its members) or a person with a mental incapacity
6 **legal purpose** (not unlawful), so that a contract to perform a criminal or other unlawful act is rendered illegal and therefore unlawful or void
7 **genuine consent** of the parties, which means the absence of factors such as misrepresentation, mistake or duress.

WHAT TO BE AWARE OF WHEN ENTERING A CONTRACT

Verbal or written representations

Care should be made in *representations* (statements about the subject matter of the contract) made prior to the contract. Such statements can become part of the contract depending upon the time the statement was made, its form and the degree of reliance on special skills or expertise of the other party. If the statement is found to be part of the contract, and the person who made the statement does not adhere to the promise made in that statement, damages for breach of contract or an action for misrepresentation may result.

For example, in relation to a contract for teaching services, a venue owner may verbally represent to a prospective teacher that the venue will, in addition to salary, allow the teacher to conduct up to 4 hours a week of lessons with his or her own students at the venue. If the teacher agrees to sign a contract (not containing details about the 4 hours of lessons) on the basis of the verbal representation, and the venue owner reneges on the promise, the teacher may have an action for breach of contract or misrepresentation.

Specifically in relation to services, the *Trade Practices Act 1974* (Cth) also makes it an offence to falsely represent:

- that services are of a particular standard, quality, value or grade
- that a particular person has agreed to acquire services
- that services have sponsorship, approval, performance characteristics, accessories, uses or benefits they do not have
- that a corporation has a sponsorship, approval or affiliation it does not have
- the price of services
- the need for any services
- the existence, exclusion or effect of any condition, warranty, guarantee, right or remedy.

For instance, if swimming lessons are promoted to the public as being 'endorsed by a high-profile Olympic swimmer' when the swimmer has not in fact endorsed them, such conduct is likely to breach the provisions of the *Trade Practices Act*.

Reduce it to writing

It is prudent for all contracts to be in written form, rather than verbal — this relieves much of the difficulty of providing evidence of the terms of the contract in the event of dispute.

The contract can be as simple as a letter outlining the relevant details and signed by both parties.

Observe the formalities

You should ensure all essential elements of offer, acceptance, consideration, intention to create legal relations, legal capacity, legal purpose and genuine consent are present.

Freedom and capacity to contract

There should be no *undue influence* in contracting — that is, no undue force or pressure should be placed on the other party to contract.

The laws applying to forming contracts with minors are complex and differ depending on the nature of the contract, and even in which state or territory the contract is made. As a general rule, a person over 18 years old may enter a binding contract, and a minor may be able to enter a binding contract in certain situations; for example if the contract is substantially for the benefit of the minor. Specialist advice should be obtained if a contract is required to be binding on a minor.

Implied terms

Certain terms will be implied into contracts by custom or by statutes — most commonly, in the sale of goods, a term is implied that the goods are of merchantable quality.

Other warranties that may be implied are that:

- services will be rendered with due care and skill
- any goods supplied with the services will be fit for the purpose
- where the purpose is made known, the services and any material supplied in connection with them will be fit for that purpose.

Therefore, no matter what a contract says, if swimming and water safety lessons are not delivered with due care and skill, a swimming teacher may be faced with a breach of contract claim from the person who has contracted the teacher to provide the swimming and water safety lessons.

Most implied terms cannot be excluded from the contract, even if the contract has an exclusion clause as discussed below.

Limitation of liability

An exclusion clause may be inserted into a contract to exclude or limit the liability of a party for breach of contract. Such a clause must be well defined, covering all bases upon which a claim might be brought and cover all those who might possibly be responsible for injury. Therefore, if a sporting organisation intends to exclude all liability including liability for negligence, then the exclusion clause should specifically state this to be the case.

Other mechanisms which can be incorporated into a contract to limit liability include *release* and *indemnity* clauses. A *release* is simply an abandonment of a right to claim. An *indemnity* is simply a transfer of the responsibility to pay for any liability from one party to the other.

A teacher of swimming and water safety should carefully read any contract he or she enters into and be aware of the effect of such clauses, which may reduce or remove any ability to recover damages in the event of a breach of contract or negligence of the other party.

Restraint of trade issues

Restraint of trade means that a restriction is placed on an employee who cannot undertake trade elsewhere in circumstances where this employment competes with their current employer. The doctrine has application to professional sport where the athlete receives reward (it even applies to part-time athletes who are paid). The courts have stated that sport is part of the entertainment industry and therefore attracts commercial principles of law such as restraint of trade.

Teachers of swimming and water safety may find they have a restraint clause in their employment contracts which prevents them from competing with their current employer for a period following termination of their employment.

A restraint of trade is not, on its face, unlawful. Every clause which seeks to restrict an employee from obtaining similar employment elsewhere is a restraint of trade. It is only where a restriction or restraint is unreasonable in the eyes of the public and not in the legitimate interest of the employer, that a court will declare the restraint as being unlawful.

CODES OF BEHAVIOUR

Where swimming and water safety teachers agree to abide by a code of behaviour, often as part of their employment, they are effectively agreeing to be bound by the provisions of the code of conduct, which operates as a contract between the teacher and the organisation which seeks to enforce it. For further information on codes of behaviour, see page 21 of this chapter and Appendix 1.

Where a teacher fails to act in accordance with a code of conduct he or she may be considered to be in breach of a contractual obligation.

SUMMARY

- A contract creates legal obligations between contracting parties.
- It is essential that any contract or agreement be produced in writing so that it is clear to the parties

as to the rights and obligations which flow from the contract.

- Care must be taken to ensure that the contract is valid and that it meets the organisation's objectives in entering the contract.
- Contracts are valuable tools which should create benefits, not be detrimental, for an organisation.
- It is recommended that swimming and water safety teachers obtain legal advice before entering into contracts.

Criminal law

Swimming and water safety teachers may be liable criminally for their actions. The criminal laws are similar in most states and territories of Australia and cover a range of conduct that society considers criminal and deserving of significant punishment. In some states and territories, it is an offence for a person to:

- do, or fail to stop, anything which causes serious danger to the life, health or safety of a person, where an ordinary person in similar circumstances would have foreseen such danger, and prevented that thing
- engage in sexual activities with a child under the age of 16 years to whom the person is not married or while that child is under the person's care, supervision or authority.

The unfortunate reality is that criminal behaviour does occur in sport. There have been numerous reported cases, particularly in the last few years, of sport administrators and officials being found criminally liable for breaches of the criminal law.

HARASSMENT/DISCRIMINATION

What is harassment?

There are a number of state, territory and federal laws that operate to prohibit harassing behaviour.

The definition of harassment adopted by the Australian Sports Commission is:

> Harassment consists of offensive, abusive, belittling or threatening behaviour directed at a person or people because of a particular characteristic of that person or people (including the person or person's level of empowerment relative to the harasser). The behaviour must be unwelcome and the sort of behaviour a reasonable person would recognise as unwelcome.
>
> (Australian Sports Commission: www.aussport.gov.au)

Whether or not the behaviour is harassment is to be determined from the point of view of the *person receiving the harassment*. The recipient must consider the behaviour to be *unwelcome*. It does not matter whether or not the person harassing intended to *offend*. The behaviour must also be assessed objectively in that it must be the type of behaviour that *a reasonable person would find unwelcome*.

SEXUAL HARASSMENT

Sexual harassment includes:

- any unwelcome sexual advance
- any unwelcome request for sexual favours
- unwelcome conduct of a sexual nature (including any statement, whether oral or written, of a sexual nature) in circumstances where a reasonable person would have anticipated that the person being harassed would be offended, humiliated or intimidated.

Sexual harassment is often, but need not be, behaviour which involves blackmail or a quid pro quo, in that the harassment is accompanied by a direct or implied threat, promise or benefit — for example, a coach who implies that a player's selection to a team is dependent on compliance with a sexual proposition.

Sexual harassment may also be a criminal offence, and can include, for example, indecent assault, rape, sex with a minor, obscene telephone calls or letters.

Another example of sexual harassment is the making of jokes or comments directed at a person's body, looks or sexual orientation.

ABUSIVE BEHAVIOUR

Abuse constitutes harassment, and includes:

- physical abuse (e.g. assault)
- emotional abuse (e.g. blackmail, repeated requests or demands)
- neglect (i.e. failure to provide the basic physical and emotional necessities of life)
- abuse of power which the harasser holds over the harassed.

People in positions of power or authority, such as a swimming and water safety teacher in relation to minors, need to be particularly wary not to exploit that power.

Many behaviours which occur in everyday sporting contexts might actually amount to a form of harassment. This may be on behalf of players, teachers, officials or spectators; for example, the encouragement of players to injure opposition team members or insults directed by students at other students.

Some forms of abuse may constitute a criminal offence; for example, assault.

Discrimination

Each state and territory has different discrimination legislation. Although there is a level of overlap, the legislation does differ. In addition, there is Commonwealth legislation which also deals with discrimination. Below is a summary of the common elements of discrimination legislation.

Discrimination is treating or proposing to treat a person less favourably than someone else in certain areas of public life on the basis of an attribute or personal characteristic they have.

These attributes or characteristics include:

- age
- disability
- marital status
- parental/carer status
- physical features
- political belief/activity
- pregnancy
- race
- religious belief/activity
- sex or gender
- sexual orientation
- transgender orientation.

Discrimination is not permitted in the following activities in which, particularly, swimming and water safety teachers may be involved:

- employment (including unpaid employment)
- the provision of goods and services
- the selection or otherwise of any person for a competition or a team
- obtaining or retaining membership (including the rights and privileges of membership).

Discrimination includes *direct discrimination* and *indirect discrimination*. Direct discrimination occurs if a person treats, or proposes to treat, someone with a particular attribute or characteristic less favourably than the person treats, or would treat, someone without that attribute or characteristic, in the same or similar circumstances.

Indirect discrimination occurs where a person imposes or intends to impose a requirement, condition or practice which on its face is not discriminatory, but has the effect of discriminating against a person(s) with a particular attribute.

Discrimination also includes *victimisation*. This is where a person is subject to, or is threatened to suffer, any detriment or unfair treatment, because that person has or intends to pursue their legal rights under anti-harassment legislation.

There are certain exceptions to discrimination which may be applicable to activities undertaken by the swimming and water safety teacher which allow discrimination in relation to the selection of a team for competition or entry to a competition, and discrimination on the basis of a person's gender is permitted if the strength, stamina and physique of the competitor is relevant.

SUMMARY

- Swimming and water safety teachers should be aware that their actions may constitute harassment in breach of the law.
- Where the person harassed is successful in a claim, they may seek monetary damages (from the person harassing them).
- Harassment may also in some circumstances constitute a breach of the criminal law which may result in fines or jail.

PRIVACY

Privacy law in Australia comprises a group of statutes and doctrines that regulate the use and disclosure by one person of information regarding another person. Generally, privacy law protects the confidentiality or secrecy of an individual's personal or sensitive information. It may also prevent a third person contacting the individual.

The key piece of legislation is the *Privacy Act 1988* (Cth) which outlines a number of National Privacy Principles which apply generally to Australian organisations and persons acting in a business capacity.

Swimming and water safety teachers often have a need to collect or use personal information in the course of their activities; for example, through membership forms or medical consent forms.

In order to avoid a breach of privacy law, they should:

- seek the consent of the person from whom the information is being collected
- only collect information for a legitimate purpose and inform the person of what the information will be used for and to whom it may be disclosed
- only use or disclose information for the 'primary purpose' for which it was collected or for a secondary purpose that the individual would reasonably expect
- ensure all information is securely stored and provide access to individuals to correct and update information that has been collected.

RISK MANAGEMENT AND IMPROVING PRACTICE

With any concept of care there is a corresponding concept of risk. In order to minimise the risks, a swimming and water safety teacher should adopt a risk management program. Risk management is a tool by which swimming and water safety teachers can seek to meet their duties and thereby limit their liability.

Risk management is a process of systematically eliminating or minimising the adverse impact of all activities which may give rise to injurious or dangerous situations. The objective is to identify, assess and control risks in order to reduce the likelihood of their occurrence and to apply effective controls to reduce the severity and consequences of those events to acceptable levels if they do occur.

Which risks need to be managed?

Importantly, the law does not require swimming and water safety teachers to provide a completely risk-free environment. Indeed, by agreeing to participate in swimming and water safety activities, participants (or their parents) will be taken to have consented to those risks which form an inevitable aspect of the activity. Teachers will not be required to take steps to counter risks where it would be unreasonable to expect a teacher to do so in the circumstances. Teachers will, however, be expected to adopt reasonable precautions against risks that might result in injuries or damages which are reasonably foreseeable.

Elements of a risk management program

The key elements of a risk management program are:
- risk identification
- risk assessment
- risk control
- monitor and review.

RISK IDENTIFICATION

The first step in a risk management program is to identify what risks exist (or may exist in the future). It is important that people who are regularly involved in swimming and water safety activities are involved in identifying risk areas. Teachers, coaches and even participants should be consulted. There is no substitute for actual practical experience in working out why accidents occur, or what presents a potential problem.

In an aquatic environment, specific risks may include risks flowing from the suitability of the surface around the water, the age or wear and tear of equipment placed around the pool or used in the lessons, and the levels of supervision in relation to the need of particular participants.

RISK ASSESSMENT

Having identified the risks involved in swimming and water safety programs and activities, you need to assess them in terms of their likelihood to occur and the seriousness of the consequences arising from their occurrence.

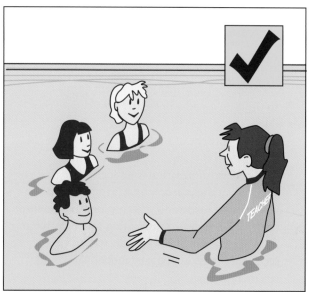

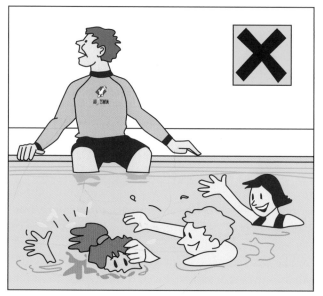

Managing risks — what are the differences here?

Each identified risk must be rated according to:

- the likelihood of the risk occurring (likelihood)
- the loss or damage impact if the risk occurred (severity)
- the priority, or degree of urgency required to address the risk.

For instance, a loose tile near the entrance to the pool may be rated highly and require immediate attention, however a loose tile against a wall in an area not used by pedestrians may be assessed as a lower risk and therefore able to be repaired at a later stage, subject to appropriate interim risk treatment.

RISK CONTROL

This stage is all about identifying and testing strategies to manage the risks that have been identified and subsequently evaluated as posing a real risk to participants. Ideally teachers will work together to brainstorm a variety of treatment strategies and then consider each strategy in terms of its effectiveness and implementation.

For instance, once you have assessed a risk you will need to carefully consider what is needed to treat the risk, who has the responsibility and what is the timeframe for risk management. These elements will constitute your action plan. If you do not have a strategy in place to address or manage an identified risk, you will have to devise a strategy.

MONITOR AND REVIEW

It is very important that teachers review the risk management plan at the end of the activity, program or term. The risk management plan should be a fluid document which is regularly updated to take account of changes within the program.

The keeping of records and the continued evaluation of the risk management plan in the light of such records is crucial. Your risk management procedures should include the documentation of any accidents, as well as information on the effectiveness of the risk management plan. Statistics on continuing injuries or accident occurrences should be used to determine whether there are specific activities that require either increased precautions or supervision.

Your risk management plan cannot remain static. Risks can change according to changes in the law, development of safer practices and techniques, and developing technology in the sport of swimming. Constant evaluation and updating must be done to take account of developing trends and the organisation's or teacher of swimming and water safety's own experience.

Communication

It is essential that all participants and parents in your programs and activities are aware of the risk management program and are consulted in its development, implementation and evaluation.

IMPLEMENTING A RISK MANAGEMENT PROGRAM

When swimming and water safety teachers are planning or implementing programs and lessons, they should identify and assess foreseeable risks and, where possible, eliminate the possibility of such risks arising in the first place. Should the risk nevertheless arise, ideally the swimming and water safety teacher should determine the way that risk is to be controlled.

The swimming and water safety teacher should:

- provide a safe environment
- plan activities with a documented lesson plan
- evaluate students or athletes for injury and incapacity
- provide safe and proper equipment
- warn students of the inherent risks of the sport
- develop clear written rules for training and general conduct
- keep adequate records
- closely supervise activities.

PLANNING FOR AN INCIDENT

A swimming and water safety teacher should be thoroughly prepared to respond appropriately should an emergency arise. Factors to be considered when planning for an emergency include:

- documentation and rehearsal of an emergency plan
- availability of rescue equipment
- a recognisable emergency signal, such as continuous blasts of a whistle
- practice of rescue techniques, including procedures for non-contact rescue and contact rescue
- capability to perform rescues in the selected teaching environment, particularly from the bottom. The availability of various aids, including fins, may improve rescue capabilities.

Examples of emergency plans and procedures are given in detail in Chapter 10, 'Plan, deliver and review a lesson'.

Consent forms

It is advisable to obtain consent forms signed by a parent or guardian/carer prior to allowing children to participate in a swimming and water safety program. It is also advisable to require a student (and the student's parent or guardian/carer if under 18) to complete a 'declaration as to fitness'. The declaration, which could form part of a consent form, should state that there is no medical or other reason why the student cannot participate in the proposed activities. A signed consent form and declaration as to fitness does not mean that a swimming and water safety teacher is immune from liability should the student be injured. However, these documents may have some weight in assisting to reduce the liability imposed upon a swimming and water safety teacher.

It is important that the information on a consent form, and declarations as to fitness are detailed enough to ensure that the student and a parent or guardian is well informed of the extent of the activity to which they are being asked to give their consent.

CONSENT FORM REQUIREMENTS
–   Aims and objectives of the program
–   Specific details of activities to be undertaken
–   Venue details
–   Program starting and finishing times
–   Transport arrangements
–   Relevant qualifications and experience of staff

The consent form (or a separate form including a declaration as to fitness) should also require the student and parent or guardian/carer to advise of any medical conditions that the student has of which the swimming and water safety teacher should be aware. Such information should also be obtained in the case of adult students.

If a student does not return a signed consent form and declaration as to fitness including their medical history, the swimming and water safety teacher may refuse to let the student participate.

When a series of similar activities takes place on a regular basis, one consent form and declaration as to fitness at the start of the series is likely to be sufficient provided the form outlines the details of the activities. It would be prudent for the actual dates over which the program is to run to be listed.

It is advisable that consent forms be translated for parents or guardians of students from language backgrounds other than English, so that they can give informed consent.

It is important to be aware that parent or guardian consent and the declaration as to fitness does not change the duty of care owed by the swimming and water safety teacher to the student.

Swimming and water safety teachers should familiarise themselves with the information provided on consent forms before commencing a program. Consent forms, together with contact numbers and relevant medical information, should be kept onsite by the pool or taken to a hired venue, to be easily accessible in case of an emergency. It is a good idea to keep them in alphabetical order.

It is also advisable that important medical information, such as who suffers from asthma, or any special requirements of particular students, are noted on student rolls so teachers are made aware at the beginning of each lesson of the risks attached to particular students. When collecting and providing information to anyone, ensure the organisation complies with the relevant privacy laws, in particular in relation to 'sensitive information', such as medical histories.

Appendix 2 is an example of a suitable consent form.

Supervision

Supervision is extremely important when children are in and around water. The swimming and water safety teacher is obligated to provide constant and active supervision as a duty of care for their students.

Teachers need to be aware that the level of supervision may need to increase depending on the age of the students, the ability of the students or the degree of risk of the activity.

Key points of supervision:

*   Constant supervision is where the teacher is no more than an 'arm's length' from students and can easily reach any student within five seconds. This is appropriate where a very high level of duty of care is applicable. For example: a group of beginners or non-swimmers.
*   A direct line of vision to all students must be maintained at all times. At no point should a teacher turn their back on the students or conduct an activity that requires students to move outside the teacher's direct line of sight.
*   Supervision must be appropriately modified when the degree of risk of an activity increases or the ability of the students decreases.
*   Students should never be left unsupervised at any time during the lesson.

Action after an incident

If a swimming and water safety teacher is unfortunate enough to be involved in a situation whereby someone is seriously injured during a lesson, it is most important that they attempt to write a report of the accident as soon as possible, while it is still fresh in their mind (see Appendix 3).

If the employer concerned has an accident report form, it should be completed and lodged, and a copy kept by the swimming and water safety teacher (see Appendix 3).

The report should be completed in ink and should contain a detailed description of what happened and what actions followed (particularly if the swimming and water safety teacher was involved in treating the injured person). If possible, it should also include the names, addresses and telephone numbers of any witnesses.

A written report and details of the witnesses are essential because court cases can often occur many years after an incident, and documentary evidence produced at the time of the incident will generally be relied on in favour of recollections or memories, which fade over time.

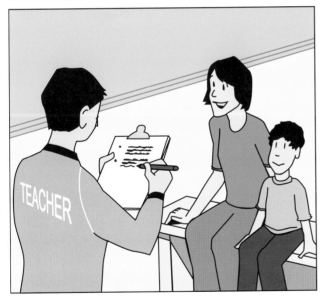

An accident report must be completed when an accident occurs during a lesson

INSURANCE

Insurance is a common risk transfer tool, in that it transfers the risk to another party (that is, to the insurer rather than the insured). It is a reactive rather than a proactive measure and swimming and water safety teachers should adopt other measures to attempt to eliminate and minimise the risk occurring in the first place. Should the risk nevertheless arise, insurance will reduce the personal liability of a swimming and water safety teacher to the extent of the cover provided.

Where a swimming and water safety teacher has insurance, it is important to know what the policy covers. For example:

- What type of incidents are covered under the policy?
- What is excluded under the policy?
- When is cover provided?
- Where is cover provided?
- What is the level of cover?

AUSTSWIM insurance cover

In order to provide protection for its swimming and water safety teachers, AUSTSWIM has arranged a group policy that can be acquired for a nominal fee once the AUSTSWIM Certificate is obtained. A copy of the insurance policy may be obtained from AUSTSWIM at www.austswim.com.au.

The main types of cover which are relevant to a swimming and water safety teacher include:

PROFESSIONAL INDEMNITY INSURANCE

This is the most relevant to a swimming and water safety teacher. Generally this type of policy covers professional people, such as swimming and water safety teachers, for legal liability where there has been error, omission or neglect by that person in the carrying out of their professional duties. Because error or neglect can lead to the person being sued for negligence, professional indemnity cover insures them against such claims. Swimming and water safety teachers should ensure that they have this type of cover either through their employer or via a private scheme.

PUBLIC LIABILITY INSURANCE

This type of policy is generally taken out by sporting organisations to protect them against claims made by a third party in respect of bodily injury or property damage arising out of the operation of the sporting organisation's business. For example, it is likely to cover a person who is injured in the course of a swimming lesson conducted by a sporting organisation.

PERSONAL ACCIDENT INSURANCE

This type of policy may be taken out by a swimming and water safety teacher. It provides cover in the form of a weekly fixed payment if a person is unable to work through sickness or accident, or in the form of a lump sum to dependants in the case of accidental death. The benefits under this policy may also include medical benefits, student assistance benefits, home help allowance and parents' inconvenience allowance.

WORKERS COMPENSATION INSURANCE

This type of insurance is taken out by employers and covers expenses such as wages and medical bills if an employee (such as a swimming and water safety teacher) is injured at work. Volunteer swimming and water safety teachers are not employees and may need additional cover under a policy for volunteer workers.

WORKING WITH CHILDREN LEGISLATION

There are mandatory responsibilities and requirements under child protection legislation for organisations and individuals that work with or have contact with children. These responsibilities apply to all teachers working with children, whether paid or voluntary.

Screening or checking processes and other requirements exist under child protection laws in each state and territory, these processes and to whom they apply, vary across states and territories.

> Further information on specific and up-to-date state/territory laws can be accessed at www.ausport.gov.au/ethics/legischild.asp.

NATURAL JUSTICE

When dealing with complaints or disciplinary matters in relation to the performance of duties of swimming and water safety teachers, it is important to treat all parties fairly and with respect. A key element of all such proceedings should be an adherence to the rules of natural justice, which will minimise the possibility of accusations of bias or unfair procedures.

The rules of natural justice can be summarised as:

- The person accused should receive notice of, and know the nature of, the accusation made against him or her. Therefore any notice should be in writing and delivered personally to the individual concerned, clearly setting out the nature, particulars and basis of the alleged breach, and clearly setting out the sanctions which may be imposed if it is determined that the alleged breach has occurred.
- The person accused should be given the opportunity to state his or her case (receive a fair hearing). This will require only relevant evidence to be considered by a tribunal or court, the corroboration of any evidence introduced, the presence of the accused in the hearing room, the opportunity for the accused to make representations, and the disclosure of all relevant facts.
- The person or body hearing the case should act in good faith and without bias. Therefore a hearing body should not pre-judge or have a financial interest in the outcome or have any conflict of interest.

These requirements will depend upon the circumstances of the case, the nature of the inquiry, the rules under which the body hearing the case is acting and the subject matter which is being dealt with. Teachers and organisations should be aware of the procedures laid down in the rules of their organisation in relation to such proceedings, which may exclude such rights as legal representation and the right to cross-examine.

In the absence of special provisions in a constitution or rules of an organisation, a person does not have to prove his or her innocence and should not be disadvantaged unless the organisation can establish a case against him or her.

AUSTSWIM TEACHER CODE OF BEHAVIOUR

As part of the AUSTSWIM registration process (Chapter 1) teachers must abide by the AUSTSWIM Teacher Code of Behaviour (refer to Appendix 1). The primary objective of the AUSTSWIM Teacher Code of Behaviour is to ensure AUSTSWIM teachers provide safe swimming and water safety programs at all times and that a high level of instruction is delivered.

CODE OF BEHAVIOUR
- Encourage public confidence in aquatic education
- Publicise AUSTSWIM's expectations of its teachers
- Show that AUSTSWIM teachers accept a standard of practice
- Provide a benchmark for appropriate behaviour

LEGAL LIABILITY — A FINAL WORD

Swimming and water safety teachers should not become paranoid about their potential legal liability. If a swimming and water safety teacher is aware of the areas in which they may be legally liable, and they address the risks which may arise in those areas, the chances of legal liability are greatly diminished.

A comparison of the thousands of hours that are spent teaching swimming and water safety throughout Australia with the number of legal proceedings brought against swimming and water safety teachers (whether for negligence or otherwise) indicates that legal liability is not a major problem for the profession at the moment. However, teachers should always keep in mind that it could happen to them, even though the chances are remote.

If swimming and water safety teachers act reasonably in the circumstances, comply with the law and adopt risk management strategies to minimise the risks arising in the first place, the chances of them being held legally liable are greatly diminished. Sports supervision is one area where risks can be substantially reduced by good housekeeping and ensuring the sporting environment is safe.

REVIEW QUESTIONS

1 What are the four areas of law that AUSTSWIM teachers need to be aware of?
2 List and explain the elements of negligence.
3 Explain how the age of a student affects the duty of care given by a teacher.
4 Explain how the following areas of law affect a teacher of swimming and water safety:
   - contract law
   - criminal law
   - harassment/discrimination
   - privacy
   - risk management.
5 What insurance cover is available to teachers of swimming and water safety?
6 What is the AUSTSWIM Teacher Code of Behaviour?

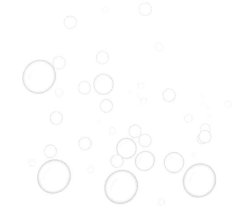

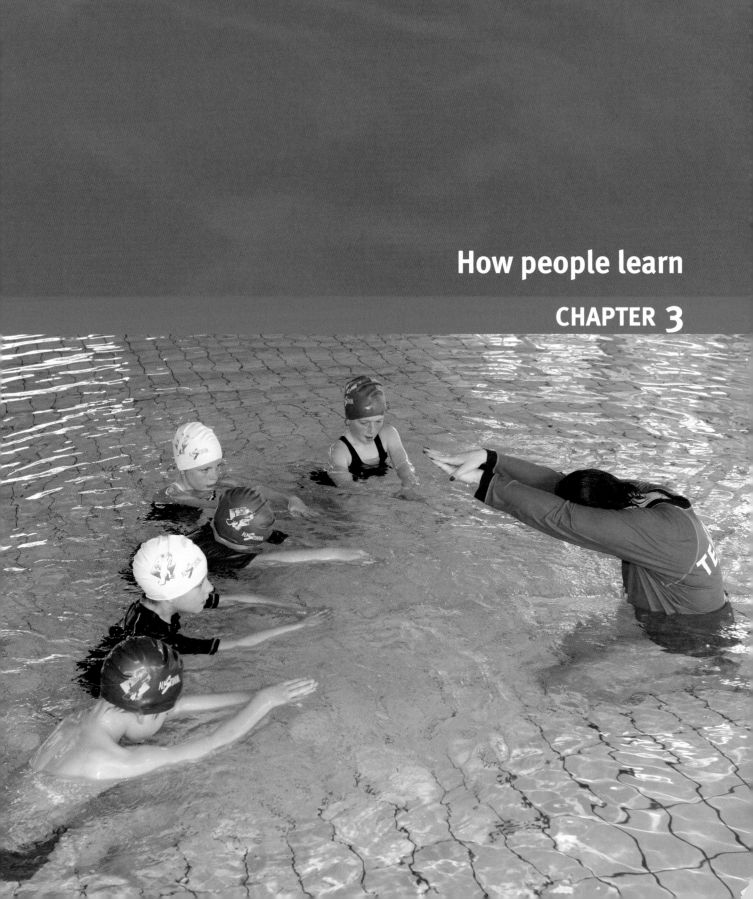

How people learn

CHAPTER 3

THE LEARNING OF SKILLS

The subject of learning, and of how learning and memory occur, has been a major topic in psychology since its birth as a scientific discipline.

In order to be an effective teacher, it is necessary to understand how people learn. It is the aim of this chapter to provide teachers of swimming and water safety with some of the basic concepts necessary to develop an understanding of how people learn motor skills. It is important to realise that learning is a continuous process that evolves over a period of time.

Learning does not necessarily take place in a formal context. Informal activities may account for much of what is learnt. Often students learn more readily from one another than from their teacher. Primarily, teachers should provide a stimulating environment in which constructive learning can take place.

Appendix 7 outlines the developmental stages of the student.

LEARNING AND PERFORMANCE

One should remember that there is a clear distinction between learning and performance. For example, a student may perform a competent stroke technique, however, unless the technique can be consistently repeated over a period of time, it cannot be said to have been learnt. This is an important factor to consider when assessing water skills — a one-off performance of skill should not be considered enough to grant a student competence. Successful teachers of swimming and water safety will take notice of their students' development over many sessions and will be able to evaluate whether the skills being taught can be performed on demand. To determine whether or not learning has taken place, teachers should analyse performances to see if there has been improvement — if this is so, they would expect to observe fewer mistakes, greater accuracy and speed, and less time taken to respond to a direction.

It should also be noted that if students have an extended break in instruction, their performance of water skills will deteriorate. This is often the case in instances where students attend lessons only for a short period each year. The ability to perform skills previously mastered will have diminished and it will be appropriate to revise those skills before progressing to more advanced techniques.

FACTORS AFFECTING SKILL PERFORMANCE

The main factors involved in learning a motor skill are discussed below.

 Environmental factors

The teacher of swimming and water safety may have to teach under varying environmental conditions, and this may adversely influence students' ability to grasp or develop the skills being taught.

ENVIRONMENTAL FACTORS TO CONSIDER
- Inside/outside teaching venues
- Weather conditions — rain, wind, cold, heat
- Water temperature
- Noise
- Nearby distractions
- The size of a teaching group
- Location — sea, river, dam or swimming pool
- Depth of water
- The amount of teaching space available

Individual factors

When teaching a skill, it should always be remembered that the whole personality of the individual is involved and that each person is unique. In a class of six students, each one will differ from the others in many respects, including physical, intellectual and emotional characteristics. These differences should be recognised and addressed in your planning and conducting of the lesson.

It is important for the AUSTSWIM teacher to acknowledge that each person brings to a class an incredible number of individual factors and to be aware that a student's behaviour might be a direct result of these. For example, people are not born knowing fear, rather it is developed through experiences. An instance of this would be a 32-year-old woman who was jammed under water (in a river) as a child and who still found it extremely difficult, years later, to duck her head under the water to collect a brick from the bottom of the pool.

TEACHING TIP
Remember that each of your students are different; plan your lesson for all of them.

Cultural background

Further to all of these individual characteristics, the culture from which the students come and their individual peer groups also contribute greatly to the manner in which they learn. In many cultures, for example, women are not allowed to have their bodies uncovered. Hence, a number need to wear full-length attire during lessons. Also, in some cultures it is not acceptable for female teachers to touch male students, as this is considered disrespectful. Teachers need to be aware of cultural differences as far as is practicable, and try to accommodate students' beliefs and values. It must be remembered, however, that safety cannot be neglected on account of these principles.

Peer group

The influence of the peer group has been well documented, and the successful AUSTSWIM teacher may be able to use it to his or her advantage. Sometimes the peer group may serve to encourage and motivate a student to attempt something when the teacher's influence cannot. Conversely, a peer group can discourage a student by, for example, laughing if a simple skill is performed poorly.

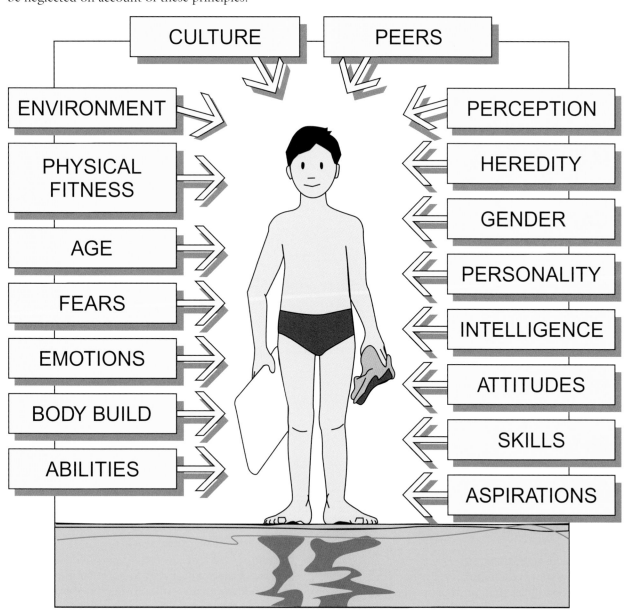

Factors affecting learning

THE LEARNING PROCESS

The theory of learning is a very complex field of study, nevertheless it is the intention of this section to outline the basic principles that affect the learning process. Important and necessary elements to be considered by teachers are:

- the learning loop
- the stages of learning
- the memory system
- effective communication.

These elements provide a theoretical basis for the teaching of motor skills.

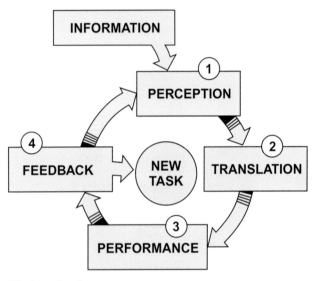

The learning loop

The learning loop

PERCEPTION

Students take in information through their sensory organs. This information is then processed and sorted in order that they may understand what it all means and decide on any action that needs to be taken. In other words, the perceptual mechanism initially interprets the information received, the brain tries to work out what it is all about, and students attempt to put it into some form of framework. Teachers can help this process by:

- providing examples appropriate to the students' experience
- using imagery or key words (recognisable to the student)
- giving demonstrations
- ensuring selective attention (for example, eliminating distractions and/or avoiding an overload of information).

TRANSLATION

The information gathered by the perceptual mechanism, and remembered because it is useful, is passed on to the translation mechanism, which obviously involves the memory system. In this decision-making stage, the student determines what to do and how to do it. One of the most important factors affecting learning is the student's understanding of what is required. Teachers can help with this stage by:

- presenting the new skill as simply as possible
- asking appropriate questions
- building on students' past experiences
- relating a new skill to something the students already know
- demonstrating the whole skill to help the students see how the parts fit together
- taking time to clarify and interpret what is required.

PERFORMANCE

When a decision has been made concerning a plan of action, students must activate the muscles which are appropriate for the response to be made. They then attempt to carry out the plan of action. Teachers can help in the performance stage by:

- providing ample opportunities for practice
- ensuring practice is regular
- making suitable use of space
- ensuring that the practice is realistic.

The importance of this last aspect cannot be overemphasised.

FEEDBACK

Feedback is an essential part of the learning process and is predominantly supplied by the teacher. Feedback can, for example, be one or more of the following:

- verbal
- visual
- written
- tactile.

Students need to obtain positive constructive feedback — that is, to be told what is wrong and how to put it right, or to be given reinforcement about what is correct.

Teachers should attempt to provide feedback as soon as possible after performance, and should avoid negative overtones. Constructive feedback is an invaluable tool in successful teaching.

Negative feedback, or knowledge of negative results, is generally considered to be 'error information' for it provides students with information about their performance and why it is not correct. If performances are to improve, it is vital to provide constructive feedback that enables students to take in new information and, if necessary, modify their action plan. The old saying 'practice makes perfect' is obviously questionable, for if students practise skills incorrectly, the skills are 'grooved' incorrectly. Practice makes permanent!

> **TEACHING TIP**
> Give feedback to your students soon after their performance and avoid negativity where possible.

The stages of learning

Skill learning is a continuous process and, as students move from being beginners to becoming more competent performers, there are three distinct stages through which they pass. The three stages are:
1 the verbal or cognitive stage
2 the intermediate or motor stage
3 the advanced or autonomous stage.

THE VERBAL OR COGNITIVE STAGE

At this stage, students try to understand the demands of the task at hand and it is important for teachers to provide them with teaching cues to which they must pay particular attention. A teaching cue provides something to look for or feel. For example, if a teacher wanted a student to obtain a high-elbow arm action in freestyle, he or she might say 'Keep your elbow high and run your fingers out along the surface of the water in line with your shoulder'. Students must be given numerous teaching cues so that they have 'indicators' that they are on the right track. They should concentrate on building up a sequence of simple skills and to this end teachers should help them to:
● recognise any previously learnt movement patterns that can be used in learning a new skill
● learn the new movement patterns that are required to perform the new skill
● integrate and arrange these two into the sequence of movements that constitute the new skill.

Here, students need only simple information in order to improve their skills. If students are overloaded with information, a correct response is unlikely. Hence, clear and concise instructions before and during practice are essential. Demonstrations should be clear to all and must be performed correctly, as students will copy what they see. Comfortable physical conditions, such as calm water of appropriate depth, warm water temperature, and a lack of disturbance from surrounding people, are necessary to achieve the most effective early learning.

> **TEACHING TIP**
> Keep the instructions simple and the demonstrations correct — your students will copy what they see.

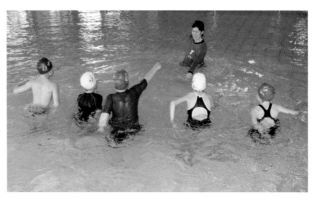

Teacher providing simple and clear instructions

THE INTERMEDIATE OR MOTOR STAGE

Students are gradually reducing the number of errors at this stage. Sometimes, when they seem to have grasped a skill, they suddenly lose it again. Teachers have to be careful, for if they apply too much pressure, students will almost certainly drop back into their old habits. During this stage teachers should try to avoid factors such as:
● asking too much too quickly
● introducing competition too early
● allowing fatigue to set in
● allowing boredom to set in.

They should remember that learning is enhanced by frequent rest periods and that at this stage the complexity of the skill governs the time involved. A number of performance improvements will begin to appear, such as:
● increased consistency in performing the skill
● improved accuracy
● decreased energy expenditure
● increased anticipation
● increased self-confidence
● improved body coordination
● increased use of motor abilities, such as flexibility, strength and speed.

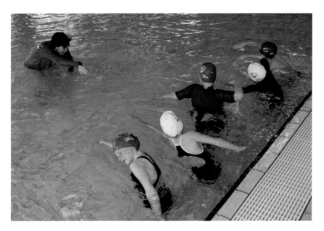

Help the students to master a skill

THE ADVANCED OR AUTONOMOUS STAGE

This is the stage where skill processes become increasingly automatic. Less processing is required and students are less affected by distractions. They are able to achieve a consistently competent level of performance. Characteristics of students at this stage are:

- their self-confidence is high
- they have a thorough understanding of the skill
- their body coordination is developed and firmly established in memory
- they can concentrate on other aspects of a skill strategy
- they are capable of evaluating their own performance.

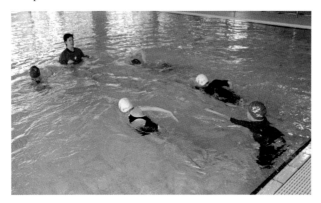

The advanced stage of learning

The memory system

Memory plays an important part in learning. Memory will either promote or inhibit the learning processes. Basically, memory is prompted by receiving a signal through the senses, which is passed into the short-term memory. The storage capacity of the short-term memory is between 1 and 30 seconds, so if the signal is not repeated, it will be lost (i.e., be forgotten).

However, if it is rehearsed it is more likely to pass into the long-term memory, which theoretically has an unlimited capacity

FACTORS AFFECTING MEMORY

Teachers must realise that a number of factors affect memory, so they must make every effort to present information in the most effective manner in order that students will retain it. Without practice, for example, students may retain about seven items (plus or minus two) in the short-term memory. After this, the information is lost. However, with practice it can be transferred to the long-term memory. To aid in this transference, teachers should:

- make the experience of learning enjoyable and fun
- provide meaningful information
- make sure the information is relevant to the students
- provide appropriate practice time in accordance with students' fitness and skill levels
- reduce distractions, such as noise
- avoid giving too much information at one time (creating overload).

CHUNKING OR GROUPING

Often teachers concentrate on individual skills and hope that students can assimilate the information on their own. However, if topics are grouped, more may be stored. This is achieved by grouping or chunking a number of related or associated items into a larger category that is more meaningful.

PROVIDING INFORMATION

Quite often, teachers feel the need to 'cram' information into students' heads. This is usually a result of:

- too little time
- too much information to present
- poor presentation.

Every individual has a certain channel capacity that can only handle a certain amount of information. In each individual this capacity will vary, but once the level is reached the student cannot absorb any more information until the previous amount has been processed. Hence, if information is given too quickly, or if too many items are given at a time, much information fails to be retained. Teachers should understand this principle and be careful to relay information at a rate appropriate for individual students.

> **TEACHING TIP**
> Remember that giving too much information at once may cause an overload for your students.

Teachers should also understand that students will focus on the most recent piece of information. Feedback relating only to the 'concentrated part' should be encouraged.

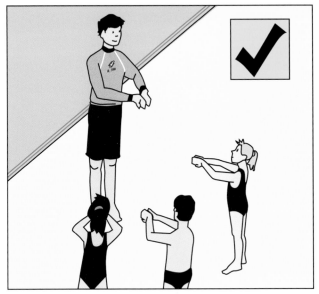

Correct way to provide information

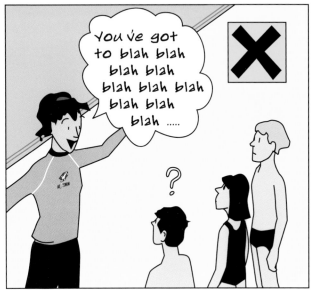

Incorrect way to provide information

Effective communication

The learning of physical skills is made easier for students if they are encouraged to:
- observe each other
- provide feedback to each other
- copy the performance of better students
- ask questions of the teacher
- ask questions of fellow students.

An all-round communication environment greatly assists with learning.

REVIEW QUESTIONS

1 List and explain the factors of learning and performance that a teacher of swimming and water safety must consider.
2 Explain the learning loop.
3 What are the three stages of learning?
4 Describe how information provided to the students by the teacher will either have a positive or negative effect.

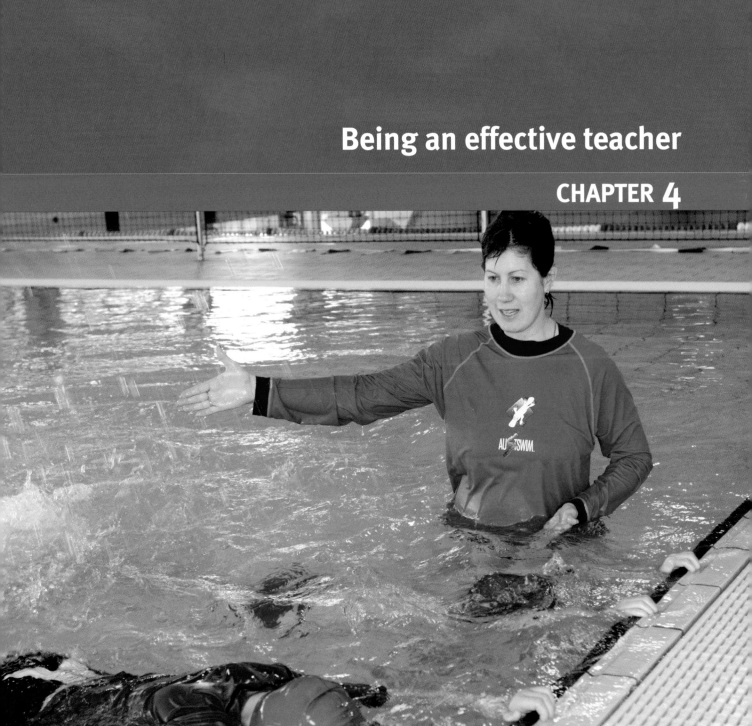

Being an effective teacher

CHAPTER 4

QUALITIES OF A GOOD TEACHER OF SWIMMING AND WATER SAFETY

What makes a good teacher? Questions about the essential characteristics of effective teaching have been at the centre of educational debates for centuries. If the answers were clear-cut, it would certainly make the task of training teachers much easier; however, some general characteristics concerning teachers and the method in which they communicate can be examined and discussed.

Good teachers are not measured just by years of experience. A successful teacher must have an open mind and a thorough knowledge of the subject, and should read widely and be ready to listen to others in order to gain more knowledge and experience.

In fact, good teachers never stop learning and are forever looking for new ideas and information.

> **TEACHING TIP**
> Remember that the mind is like a parachute — it works best when it is open.

 ## Promoting swimming and water safety

Although the learning of the physical skills related to swimming and water safety is critical, great attention also must be paid to the positive attitudes and feelings that a good teacher develops in each student (and observer). A good teacher will maintain and project a clear understanding of the benefits to be derived from 'enjoying water'.

Such a teacher will be a positive role model for all concerned, will express and display the pleasures that water offers and will continually promote the benefits of aquatic education and participation.

In particular, teachers of both young and not-so-young students should not underestimate the influence they may have on the lifelong attitude of those in their care.

Professional presentation

The teacher should appear responsible, efficient and cheerfully confident. Employers generally seek staff who demonstrate these qualities. AUSTSWIM teachers' responsibility for promoting the importance of swimming and water safety can be undermined if

they appear too casual, timid or careless; the way they look undoubtedly has an effect on the people they teach. Also, teachers must always be suitably attired to teach in the water (e.g. rash vest, appropriate swimwear, hat for outdoors).

 ## Fostering positive student relationships

Teachers should endeavour to learn and use the names of students and try to speak to each one regularly during a lesson. By doing this, they demonstrate their interest in each person.

A major part of a good relationship will be trust. Students must learn to trust their teachers and it is incumbent on the teachers to foster and develop this trust. Students are going to be asked, for example, to sit on the bottom of the pool, open their eyes under water, dive into deep water or recover an object from the pool floor — all activities that require trust in the person directing them. Students can be 'encouraged' into activities, but if at any time they discover this has been done then the trust element is lost — maybe forever.

 ## Competent organisational skills

Teachers are professional people, and the manner in which they present their work should reflect this. Lesson planning and the selection and placement of suitable teaching, swimming and rescue aids should be completed prior to the commencement of each session. However, it is important to remember that lesson planning provides only a framework in which to operate. Teachers must be able to adapt to unexpected circumstances; they must be alert to the changing dynamics of the class and cater for them. Particularly in an aquatic environment, they must function calmly and efficiently in all teaching situations and conditions, being alert and flexible at all times.

 ## Ability to inspire confidence

Beginner students often lack confidence when in the water, and in their own abilities. Teachers must use positive reinforcement to inspire confidence, and this can be done by managing the class confidently and by giving correct and efficient assistance. Teachers must establish a cooperative working spirit with the class and between the students, using appropriate assertive techniques in all aspects of class management.

Maintaining class control

For the inexperienced teacher, this may seem like a simple, obvious and automatic facet of teaching. However, closer examination reveals that to maintain class control is anything but easy. There are many variables that can place heavy demands on the teacher's ability to control a class. Factors such as class size, pool space, deep or shallow water, surrounding noise levels, the general public, other classes and limited equipment can all be disrupting elements for both teachers and students. Teachers must maintain a smooth flow of activity while communicating effectively with both individuals and groups, according to the ability of the students.

Discipline

Discipline is necessary to ensure safety and to create a satisfactory learning environment. When in the water the class should learn to stand still, look at the teacher and be quiet while explanations are given. If this control is established early, discipline problems should not arise. If a class is difficult, the teacher needs to consider whether this is due to boredom because instructions are too long, the task is either too difficult or too easy, or because the students do not understand the instructions given. Promises that cannot be kept and threats that cannot be enforced should be avoided, or respect will soon be lost.

Selecting class formations that maximise participation and do not cause students to wait for turns will leave no time for them to devise their own amusement.

If all avenues of discipline have been attempted and a student is still uncooperative and requires an unacceptable amount of individual attention, it may be prudent to decide that he or she should not be permitted to continue taking part in the current activity. After a suitable period has elapsed, the student may be allowed to once again participate.

A sense of humour

Possessing a sense of humour is always a distinct advantage, and never more so than when you are teaching. It is very important to share experiences with students; most of these experiences will be enjoyable and some will be funny. Having a good sense of humour will allow teachers and students to benefit from these moments. On the other hand, at no time should laughing at someone else's expense occur.

Enthusiasm

Students who have enjoyed their learning experiences probably had enthusiastic, encouraging teachers. Certainly, sometimes it is very difficult to be enthusiastic, particularly if the lesson is the sixth for the day in a humid, stuffy environment and it is nearly time to go home. However, it is important to remember that for the members of the class it is probably their only swimming and water safety lesson for the day and they have been looking forward to it. They expect and should receive a lively, motivating, encouraging, enthusiastic teacher to guide them successfully in their aquatic experiences.

> **TEACHING TIP**
> Be enthusiastic! You may have had a long day but your students are only with you for a short period of time each class.

Ability to demonstrate

Should a teacher be able to perform a skill in order to teach it? This question has been argued for many years.

An examination of swimming coaches would indicate that the answer to this question is 'No'. Many swimming coaches would not be able to perform a skill to the same level or ability as can the people they are coaching. What they can do, very successfully, is break the skill/activity down into logical, progressive stages, so that the swimmers can master each level. It is also a big advantage if they can demonstrate the skill — in situations where this is not possible a teacher might ask the best student or another skilled performer to provide the demonstration.

Nevertheless, as it is important for teachers to know what it is they are asking of their students, prior experience would be advantageous.

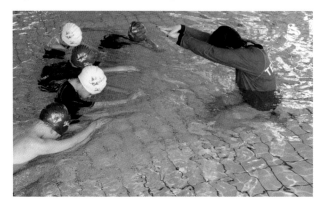

Using demonstrations

Thorough knowledge of subject

Skilled teachers need knowledge of their specialist areas as well as the theory of the learning process. They should be able to communicate well at the appropriate level and provide encouragement by a diversity of methods. Before sound teaching can take place, they need to understand what affects learning; therefore, the teacher must understand the skills to be taught, the sequential skill progressions and the causes of common faults so that corrections can be made.

Supervision and observation at all times

It is through observation that the successful teacher assesses the moods, attributes, needs and potential of both individuals and groups. Moreover, since the aquatic teaching area is potentially a dangerous one, teachers must be alert and use their 'senses' in and around the water to ensure a safe environment. They must keep an eye out for hazards and constantly take mental note of where each student is performing; for example, one may be drifting into deep water or into the path of lap swimmers. If underwater or deep water activities are being conducted, observation and supervision must be increased. If four students submerge, four students must surface! And the teacher must be the last person to leave the teaching area, after ensuring that every student is safely out. In no circumstances should a teacher leave students unattended for any amount of time.

An effective teacher will also possess a trained eye that can observe and analyse technical performance; correct positioning in order to observe a specific aspect of a stroke performance or activity is critical.

Safety is paramount in any aquatic program; it overrides everything else! Chapter 5 deals with aquatic safety essentials in detail.

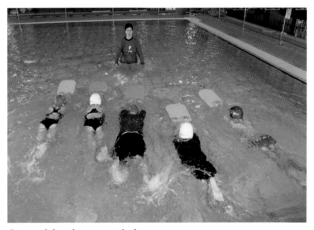

Supervision is extremely important

Recognising the teachable moment

While observation of individual students is vital, general observation throughout the lesson is the means by which teachers can determine the achievements and understanding of the class as well as note possible movement progressions. Often teachers may be looking for those whose response to a challenge is worth sharing or showing to the rest of the class. This creates what is often referred to as a 'teachable moment': the teacher has an opportunity to develop knowledge and understanding by utilising student response. Teachers should seize upon this moment to enhance learning.

Patience and understanding

A key factor in successful teaching is patience. Students should not be rushed through progressions in order to satisfy a time schedule. Rushing through practices and activities will only serve to inhibit the learning rate and detract from the enjoyment of learning to swim. Students must be encouraged to work at their own pace and to gain a range of positive experiences that will enhance their learning. People need time for information to sink in, and this is particularly true for beginners. Teachers must take this into consideration when planning their lessons.

Effective communication skills

Perhaps the most critical of skills that enhance the effectiveness of a teacher of swimming and water safety is the ability to communicate. Teachers need to communicate in a style appropriate to the person's age and sensory or intellectual impairment (e.g. sensory loss or hearing loss).

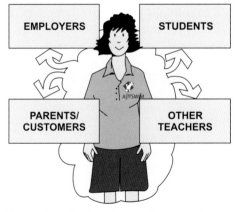

Who will a teacher of swimming and water safety need to communicate with?

COMMUNICATION WITH STUDENTS

Communication in this respect is based upon following the three Cs:

1 clarity
2 conciseness
3 consistency.

Clarity

People communicate by sight (via expressions and demonstrations) as well as by sound (through language).

A teacher should avoid ambiguous expressions and always use positive reinforcers, such as a friendly smile on greeting, or in recognition of an improved performance. Performance demonstrations must be correct, and be clearly visible to all students.

Teachers sometimes forget to consider the experience level of the students; it is important to speak at an appropriate level that avoids talking either up to or down to the class. An example of this is in the use of the word 'turbulent' or 'choppy' when speaking to primary school children. 'Turbulent' can be used effectively for discussion at teenage or adult levels, but is usually beyond the comprehension of most primary school children; an appropriate word to use at the younger child's level would be 'choppy', even though it is not as precise. Another example might be to say 'Blow bubbles' to primary school children, rather than 'exhale'.

Conciseness

Unfortunately, many teachers are prone to verbosity. Talking excessively may initially be a cover for nervousness or lack of experience, but it can develop into a bad habit.

Lengthy instructions are wasted; only short items of information will be extracted from the total. Try to give a brief positive instruction for the action to be performed, so that confusion is minimised; for example, 'Blow bubbles into the water' is a brief, positive statement, whereas 'Don't hold your breath' is negative, and the student may not hear the 'don't' and think 'What a good idea! Never thought of that!' and hold their breath! It is much better to give a short explanation, allow students to practise and then follow up with a further short explanation.

TEACHING TIP
Keep instructions brief and avoid negative statements.

Consistency

Consistency applies to both behaviour and language. Teachers are individuals too, but should try to control extremes of behaviour caused by non-teaching factors, such as tiredness after a late night, which can result in a lack of patience. This does not mean that a teacher must avoid displaying individual behaviour such as the expression of approval or disapproval, but only that the level of reaction should be a reflection of the level of behaviour that caused it.

A lack of language consistency can be a problem in the use of both normal and technical language. With the former, teachers should use descriptions that avoid extremes — such as 'fantastic' — because a later performance that might be much better could not receive an appropriate increase in praise. It is akin to achieving a score of 10 in gymnastics — where do we go from here? Teachers should also try to reflect a consistent, positive attitude in the language used. Negative words such as 'bad' or 'poor' should be avoided where possible.

Voice control

The voice level should be sufficient to reach all students clearly, without disturbing others around the pool. The volume should be lowered if students are nearby and raised if they move away. Shouting and yelling down a lane or across the pool should be avoided, not only is it very disruptive, it also adds to an already noisy environment and does little to create a safe working and learning environment. Protect your throat and reduce your stress levels by speaking slowly and clearly. Add the use of visual cues; for example, pointing to the ear while saying 'Keep the ear flat when turning to breathe', or pointing to the knees when explaining the importance of keeping them below the surface in backstroke, can develop an association of ideas whereby the student needs only visual cues.

Visual cues

Many people have difficulty hearing when they are in the water. This may be caused by deafness, water in the ears or the use of bathing caps or ear plugs. It is recommended to use visual guides in the form of hand signals to aid communication. If there are several teachers in the pool area, this can also help to reduce the general noise level; for example, if students have swum out several metres then hand signals can indicate the method of return and beckon them back. Other visual cues include pointing to a high elbow; demonstrating flutter kick using the hands, or demonstrating the arm recovery action in backstroke.

Verbal instructions

Individual instructions should begin with the student's name; for example: 'Monica, roll your head to the side to breathe, not your hips'. If the name is mentioned last, the message is finished before Monica becomes aware that it was directed to her. Also, only one or two teaching points should be given at a time.

When sending students across the pool, the teacher should be sure to watch them finish or they may think 'Nobody even saw me!' Then, instead of just the instruction 'Swim back', at least one positive teaching point should be given.

COMMUNICATING WITH PARENTS OR CUSTOMERS

When working with young students, teachers should inform parents about:

- the program philosophy and outline
- methods by which they can assist their child to master the appropriate skills
- ways of encouraging their 'little champion'
- the overall aims and objectives of the program
- progressive achievement
- the positive personal characteristics of their child.

In all programs (commercial and non-commercial), it is essential that a customer service plan includes regular formal and informal communication with students, parents and carers.

COMMUNICATING WITH EMPLOYERS

Teachers instructing students in swimming and water safety are faced with key expectations from their employers, who require positive results. A teacher needs to understand the outcomes desired by the employer, the level of professionalism required and the procedures established for dealing with difficulties that arise.

The only sure way to ensure that the expectations of employers are being met is to communicate with them both formally and informally. Teachers should continually seek advice, assistance and information from employers in order to avoid misunderstandings or communication breakdown.

It is also essential to be loyal to all involved in the aquatic industry — the employer, fellow teachers, the parents and students — and to avoid making disparaging comments about others.

COMMUNICATING WITH FELLOW TEACHERS (PEERS)

A friendly, supportive and collaborative teaching environment promotes a happy, harmonious and professional learning atmosphere. An effective teacher of swimming and water safety will offer advice to — and seek feedback from — their peers. Through adopting a collaborative approach to planning, teaching and evaluating, teachers develop a team approach that provides opportunities to continue learning and updating knowledge and ideas.

Similarly, a collaborative and united teaching team offers support to individual members in times of difficulty and also provides a forum for good teaching to be recognised and acknowledged through regular formal and informal feedback from colleagues.

TEACHING METHODS

Teaching methods refer to the way the teacher presents learning experiences.

Teachers can and should make use of a variety of styles and methods; no one style will work with all students, there is no one magical way to teach, and anyone who claims that there is has become blinkered, and his or her teaching effectiveness will be lessened. Some learning situations lend themselves to the use of a lecture style, others to the repetition of drills, while others will permit a less guided approach, where the student is confronted with problems to solve and discuss. Some students will respond better to drills; others learn best when they are challenged to solve problems. Teaching methods vary along a continuum from command to discovery.

 The whole-skill strategy

This strategy focuses on attempting a simple skill without using back-up progressions. After examination of the skill presentation, and through careful activity selection, practice and feedback, the teacher refines and improves the skill performances of the student.

 The progressive-part strategy

This involves the teacher selecting and progressively presenting various parts that culminate in the learning of the skill. Most teachers use this approach for complex skills.

As a general rule, one should not proceed from one skill to the next until the current task is well mastered. However, there are situations when one should not persist too long and it is wise to move to another skill, perhaps retracing the abandoned step later. Flexibility in teaching is knowing when to move on and when to repeat.

The whole-skill/progressive-part strategy

This is a combination of the previous two strategies that is used for both simple and complex skills. The whole skill is attempted first to enable the teacher to recognise starting points for a progressive sequence of activities designed to facilitate learning. This will also provide a framework to which the student may relate when practising the component parts.

Demonstration

As has been stated, the teacher must ensure that the whole class can clearly see a demonstration. They should not, for example, be looking into the sun, and they may need to be out of the water while the teacher (or demonstrator) is in it. But be wary of the effects of cool breezes on wet bodies out of water!

Remember that a very high percentage of information enters the brain by way of students' visual senses; therefore, what they see, they tend to copy. For this reason it is important to provide them with the best demonstration possible. To achieve the highest rate of learning from this strategy, teachers should ensure that students:

- watch the demonstration attentively
- understand what is wanted of them
- have the ability to perform the skill
- are motivated
- are focused on a small number of points
- are well organised, to avoid distractions
- are exposed to the correct techniques.

> **TEACHING TIP**
> Students learn mainly from things they see, therefore good use of demonstrations are important.

Command teaching

This involves directing the student to perform very specific tasks. It may take the form of demonstrating the task for the class to emulate, or verbally directing a class through a series of progressive drills that culminate in the performance of the final task. When time is limited, this can be a very efficient method of maximising the number of practices that can be completed.

Problem solving and discovery

These methods set tasks for the students to examine and discuss, then attempt to develop suitable responses. They rely on the teacher being able to gradually modify or shape the student's response towards the skill or knowledge goal.

Class formations

There are several different formations commonly used with swimming and water safety classes. The position of the teacher in relation to the class will vary according to the following factors:

- climatic elements, such as wind and sun
- distracting factors within the class's sight or hearing
- whether the teaching area is natural or constructed
- the skill being taught
- the age and skill of the student.

The overriding consideration must be the safety of the student.

SEMICIRCLE

A semicircle formation ensures that each student can see and be seen by the teacher.

Legend

■ Student

● Teacher

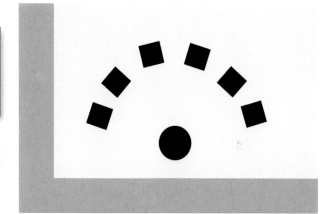

Semicircle class formation

INFORMAL

This formation ensures that all can see and be seen by the teacher, but there is less formality. It may be necessary to see that each student allows enough space between themselves and the next student to practise the required skill safely.

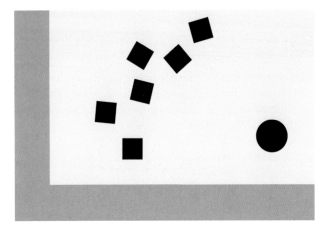

Informal class formation

LINES

Lines are used when all students are to practise at the same time. Parallel lines are used in paired activities.

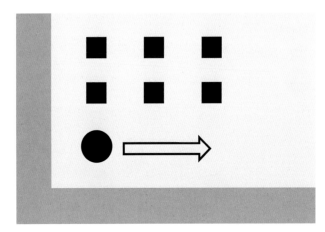

Line class formation

USE OF THE CORNER

The corner formation can be used for a variety of teaching situations. It can ensure that all students can clearly see the demonstration of a stationary skill, such as treading water in deep water. It can also be used for beginners as it allows for different activities to be incorporated within the one group. The distance of this pattern can be adjusted according to students' abilities, allowing for independent mobility while maintaining close teacher contact.

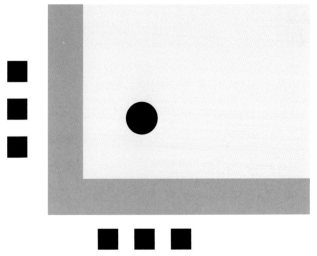

Corner class formation (students can be in or out of the water)

WAVE

This is a versatile practice formation. Students line up a comfortable distance apart and begin the activity at the same time and at their own pace.

The distance out to the teacher should be kept short to ensure a lot of repetitions but to also guard against over-working the students. Students must not be permitted to move beyond the teacher.

A variation to the standard wave formation is the 'staggered wave'. A staggered wave is used for repetition practices; the teacher can move along the group and provide individual help while the students continue practising.

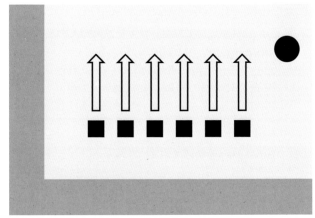

Wave class formation

CIRCLE FORMATIONS

Circle swimming may be used to provide varying distances to cater for the different capabilities of the students.

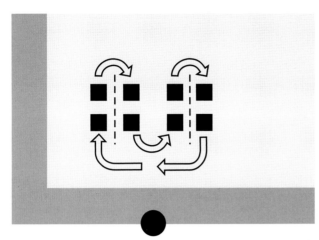

Circle class formation (teacher can be in or out of the water)

TRIANGLE

This pattern is good for the advanced student to encourage them to move away from the security of solid walls and for working over greater distances.

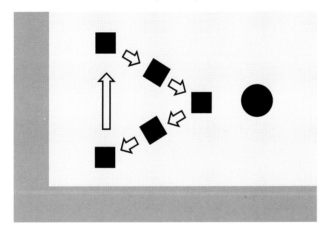

Triangle class formation

TEACHING TIPS

With any type of class formation:
- the teacher has a clear view of all students at all times
- the teacher has contact with all students and is able to give encouragement and offer corrections
- the distance is increased as skills and confidence increase.

HELPFUL TEACHING HINTS

- Be aware of safety requirements at all times.
- Be punctual in both starting and finishing; only then can you expect the same from your group.
- Prepare your work thoroughly. Don't be afraid to use a palm card as a memory aid.
- Place yourself where you can observe all the students and where all of them can see you.
- Don't try to shout to make yourself heard above noise; wait for quiet and then proceed. Bring the group closer, if necessary. Speak clearly and concisely.
- Demand full attention and immediate response to directions.
- Generally assemble groups in position for an activity before giving an explanation or demonstration.
- When teaching new work, first direct attention to the major features.
- Don't talk too much. Place the emphasis on the activity. Most people find it difficult to remember a lot of details.
- Differentiate between idle chatter and the noise of people at play.
- Use hand signals to avoid straining the voice.
- Enforce rigidly whatever rules are necessary (possibly the fewer rules the better).
- Be tactful and fair.
- Keep all students as busy as possible.
- Avoid dead spots or long breaks from activity. Make use of fun skill-based activities to enhance a teaching point.
- Don't introduce too much new work in the one session. Repetition of previous work is not only advisable, but essential for development of a satisfactory standard of performance.
- Make use of the competitive element, but don't overdo it. Try to develop the attitude that competing is better than winning.
- Provide variety in the program to cater to all tastes.
- Show care and respect for equipment and develop a routine for handling it. This is one definite way to eliminate waste of time and money.
- Delegate responsibility and develop leadership within the group.
- Make the lesson live, and become part of it. Be master of the situation, but develop the correct balance between aloofness on the one hand and over-interaction at the group level on the other.

REVIEW QUESTIONS

1 List the qualities of an effective teacher.
2 Explain the importance of communication and who a teacher would regularly communicate with.
3 Describe how different teaching methods can be used to effectively communicate information.
4 List and describe the different class formations a teacher can utilise.

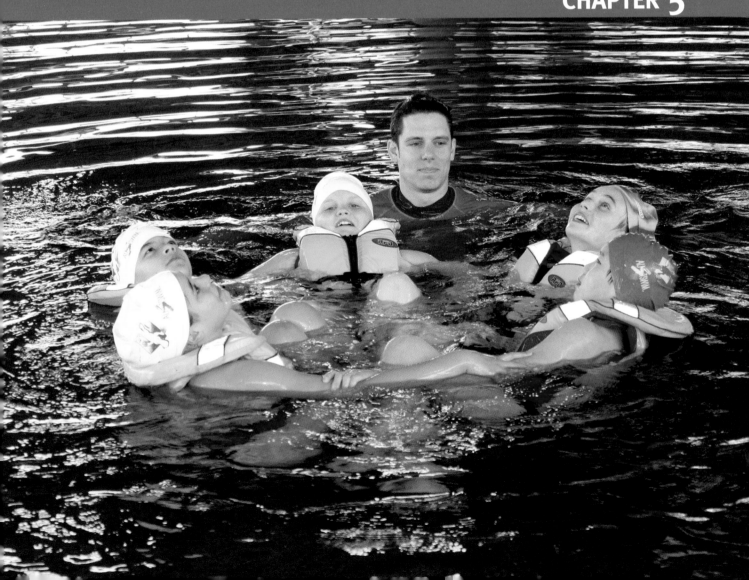

Aquatic safety, survival and rescue skills

CHAPTER 5

AQUATIC SAFETY

 Introduction

Adults placed in a position of authority have a 'duty of care' to those in their charge.

The AUSTSWIM Teacher of Swimming and Water Safety award is a qualification for the accreditation of teachers of swimming and water safety. (It is not a rescue qualification.) As a requirement of the AUSTSWIM course, candidates undergo a practical assessment of water safety, survival and rescue skills considered applicable for teaching in enclosed water environments of limited depth. The assessment indicates each candidate's ability to use those rescue skills, on that day, under limited conditions, and within recommended student–teacher ratios (see the AUSTSWIM policy on student–teacher ratios). The skills required to perform a rescue in more demanding environments (e.g. deep or open water) are far more complex and require additional training.

Employers are responsible for ensuring that the teachers they employ are competent in the essential rescue skills that are appropriate for the environment in which they are teaching.

Both the Royal Life Saving Society Australia (RLSSA) and the Surf Life Saving Association (SLSA) have informative lifesaving training manuals and award programs.

This chapter aims to provide essential water safety knowledge that should be an integral part of a swimming program and rescue skills that may be required by teachers. Safety is the highest priority in any aquatic activity. This chapter will assist teachers to conduct all lessons safely and to impart knowledge to their students for their own personal aquatic safety.

Water safety education

Water safety is an essential component of every aquatics program. For children, water safety education should begin at home in the very early years. It is important that this education should continue throughout the aquatics program.

Water safety education is not confined to formal education programs but should be combined with aquatic skill development. It reaches the broader community through awareness campaigns in newspapers, television announcements and advisory signs at popular aquatic locations, which in many cases are in English as well as languages other than

English to assist international visitors and those from Australia's multicultural population.

Advisory signs, in both natural environments and public swimming pools, warn venue users of the dangers associated with the particular environment and explain how to obtain assistance in an emergency. On piers, jetties and some rock-fishing locations, warning signs are accompanied by rescue equipment and instructions for its use.

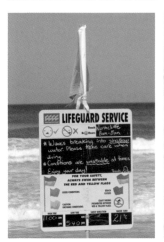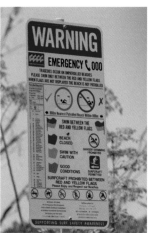

Advisory signs

The aim of water safety education is to enable students to recognise and assess potential aquatic dangers and to develop a realistic understanding of their swimming ability in various water and weather conditions. The practice of water safety, lifesaving and survival skills should commence early in the aquatic program within the constraints of the pool environment. As confidence and ability increase, these skills should be practised in open water if at all possible. The students will develop confidence, competence, endurance and judgment skills that should maximise the chance of survival in an emergency.

Water safety education is primarily concerned with the prevention of drowning. By using the skills learnt in the program and by acknowledging the importance of self-preservation, students should be able to avoid life-threatening situations. However, some emergency incidents are not predictable and the ability to make a calm assessment and to perform survival skills suitable to the particular conditions are essential.

Drowning statistics

Unfortunately a number of drownings occur each year in Australia despite the availability of water safety education programs and the number of public awareness campaigns that are conducted. While the number of drowning deaths is decreasing, there are still people who drown in common circumstances each year.

The RLSSA conducts research of aquatic incidents and drowning in Australia in order to better understand the associated factors and trends. The statistics indicate that:

- 80% of those who drown are male
- the 0–5 age group has the highest rate of drowning deaths of any age group in Australia
- drowning deaths occur across all types of locations; for example, bathtubs, pools, lakes, dams, rivers, beaches
- while the majority of people drown while undertaking aquatic activities, there are a number who end up in the water when they were not prepared
- every year a number of people drown while attempting to rescue another person.

Every year the RLSSA produces a report examining drownings for the previous 12 months. The *National Drowning Report* is available at www.royallifesaving. com.au.

Hazards of aquatic environments

The dangers inherent in an aquatic environment stem from a number of factors, including physical features, the types of water and the ability and activity of the user.

THE HOME ENVIRONMENT

The home may have potential aquatic dangers, particularly for adventurous young children who have little or no fear of the water. Those responsible for their supervision may be momentarily distracted by a ringing telephone or a knock at the door, and during this brief time a child may drown. Potential dangers around the home include:

- unfenced swimming pools or gates left open
- farm dams and water troughs
- fishponds or water features
- domestic bathtubs and spas
- washing tubs and machines
- buckets filled with liquids
- filled paddling pools
- eskies with melted ice
- toilets.

Young children must be constantly supervised by adults — that is, within arm's reach — whenever they are near water, even during bath time. In addition to supervision, it is recommended to take the following precautions:

- install a safety barrier around home swimming pools and spas with a self-closing and self-latching gate according to the Australian Standard AS1926 (as per many state and territory laws)
- empty baths, buckets, eskies, basins, sinks and troughs immediately after use
- keep plugs out of reach of young children
- securely cover liquid-filled buckets and basins, or keep them out of the reach of children
- empty children's paddling pools when they are not in use
- close top-loading washing machines
- install a mesh cover over fishponds and water features
- install rigid covers over spas
- always stay with children at bath time.

SUPERVISE CHILDREN AT ALL TIMES WHEN IN, ON OR AROUND WATER

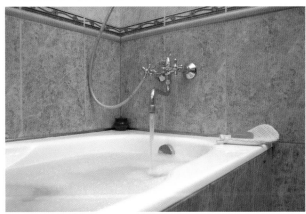

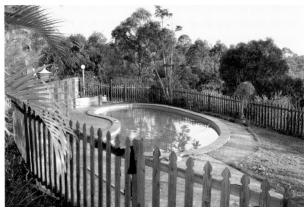

Potential hazard sites at the home

FARMS

On farms there are many bodies of water including dams, irrigation channels, water troughs, post holes and water tanks, all of which make farms potentially dangerous environments. Hazards include steep and slippery banks, deep water, strong currents due to pumps, and cold water.

To ensure safety at all times the following measures are recommended:

- create a child-safe play area near the home where children can be supervised by an adult — the safe play area should not be in the vicinity of water bodies
- nominate a designated safe area for swimming and always go with a friend
- enter the water slowly and safely to check the conditions of the bottom
- check for any hazards before entering the water such as obstacles.

TEACHING TIP

Always tell your students to check for hazards before entering any body of water.

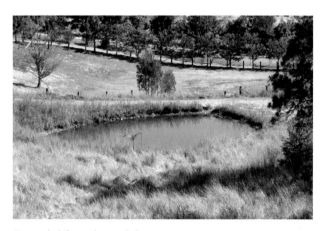

Potential farm hazard site

PUBLIC SWIMMING POOLS

Public swimming pools are usually supervised by lifeguards, whose role it is to ensure the safe operation and function of the facility. They cannot supervise every individual in a facilty. This is the role of accompanying adults, including teachers, parents and carers. However, accidents still occur, so users should consider the following advice:

- read and obey notices
- follow the instructions of lifeguards
- ensure that the water depth is appropriate for swimming or diving
- if a weak swimmer, stay away from deep water
- check that the water is clear before jumping or diving
- play safely and do not hinder the enjoyment of other users.

RIVERS, LAKES AND DAMS

A river has a continuous and often fast current that, when combined with submerged logs, overhanging branches and other obstacles, can create extremely dangerous situations.

The level of a river may change considerably over a period owing to increased rainfall in surrounding watershed areas, increased release of water for irrigation purposes and/or tidal changes. Also, the river bed itself can change rapidly and considerably following periods of heavy rain, upstream flooding and/or releases of dam water.

The current on the outside of a bend in a meandering river is usually much faster than that on the inside. Consequently, silt is likely to be deposited on the inside curve, creating an area of shallow water that is potentially dangerous because of its soft, unsupportive base. Holes often form in the soft sand and are hazardous because of the sudden change in depth.

Extreme care should always be taken when entering rivers because of their changeable nature. In no circumstances should anyone dive into a river without carefully checking the depth and possible underwater hazards.

Lakes and dams may present a deceptively still, flat appearance that can promote a false sense of security; however, conditions may change rapidly with the onset of strong winds.

Feeder rivers create unexpected, strong currents, which may take a swimmer away from the edge. Also, as these currents abate silt is dropped, forming a soft, uneven and unsupportive base.

High-altitude lakes, deep lakes and those fed by mountain streams are often very cold all year round. As a result, anyone who is immersed for a period can become stressed. Dams also contain 'cold spots', and the mud around the edges is usually very slippery, soft and difficult to move across.

Waves on lakes and dams are usually moderate in size, but they are often close together and can be difficult to swim past when they have broken. Managing craft such as canoes and kayaks in these conditions is very difficult.

The following observations are important if preparing to swim in a river, a lake or a dam:

- check with local residents on the condition of local waterways
- be aware of weather conditions and be alert for sudden change
- never swim alone
- only participate in aquatic activities, such as water skiing, in designated areas
- be careful not to stand on overhanging banks

- before entering the water, check for the presence and strength of a current
- if caught in a fast river current, travel feet first in order to absorb any impact with the feet and legs, thus protecting the head and body from serious injury
- if drawn over a weir, immediately dive to the bottom, tuck into a ball and hold breath until thrown to the surface
- before attempting to dive, check the depth and explore the bottom to locate any trees, logs, snags, sandbanks, weeds, rocks or other hazards
- enter cold water slowly and remain in for only short periods.

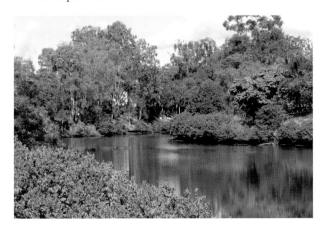

Rivers are potential hazard sites

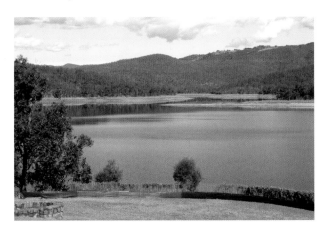

Lakes are potential hazard sites

WATER CROSSINGS

Drownings have occurred at water crossings mainly during periods of flooding, when the water has risen quickly and is moving swiftly. During these times it is important to remember:

- do not cross flowing water
- heed all warnings issued by local authorities
- observe water level indicators at low-water crossings

- road surfaces may have been washed away
- vehicles can easily stall in water and be carried away
- be extremely vigilant when travelling on unfamiliar roads or at night.

THE SEA

The movement of the sea, the height and strength of waves, the direction of currents, the tides and rips are all constantly changing. Even bay and harbour beaches, which are usually protected and are therefore considered to be less hazardous than ocean beaches, can present real dangers under certain weather conditions.

When beyond standing depth in the sea, it is a constant and sometimes strenuous effort to remain afloat and to repeatedly dive under large waves.

Swimmers at the beach should:

- stay between the red-and-yellow flags, because this area is patrolled by lifeguards
- leave the water if they are starting to feel cold
- never swim alone — always swim with another person
- not enter the water if there are any doubts regarding ability to cope with the conditions
- use surfboards, wave skis or boogie boards (with fins) only in designated areas
- read warning signs and act accordingly.

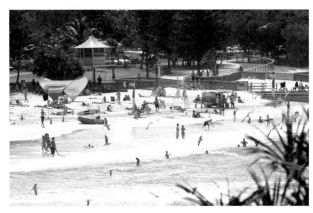

Beaches contain many hazards

Plunging waves

Plunging waves, commonly called dumpers, break with tremendous force and a swimmer can easily be thrown to the ocean floor and sustain injury. If caught in a dumper, the swimmer should assume the tuck position, protect the face with the hands and forearms and roll with the wave until it has passed.

Spilling waves

Spilling waves are safe for swimmers, body surfers and board riders. This formation occurs when the crest tumbles down the face of the wave.

Surging waves

Surging waves occur where the shoreline immediately drops into deep water; for example, where the beach is very steep or at the edge of rocky foreshores. These waves may never break as they approach and as a result there is a sudden unexpected surge of water on the beach. The consequent increase in depth and the subsequent undertow created by the receding water may cause a person standing at the water's edge to lose balance and be washed into the sea.

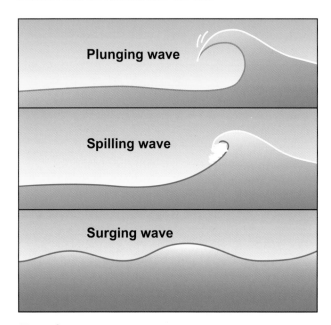

Types of waves

Rip current

A rip is deceptive as the water appears very calm, however, a rip current is a body of water moving rapidly out to sea and is a major reason behind sea rescues. It is formed by water seeking its natural level following a build-up near the beach, which is caused by large waves. The rip current forms when the retreating water concentrates in a channel. The larger the surf, the more intense will be the rip current. Sand bars often build up adjacent to rip currents.

Rip currents can be recognised by:
- the rippled appearance of the water
- waves breaking on each side of a relatively calm channel
- discolouration due to sand particles carried in the water
- debris being carried out to sea.

Rips are obvious sources of danger. Swimmers caught in a rip should float until the current weakens and then swim parallel to the shore until reaching an area where the waves are moving towards the shore and breaking.

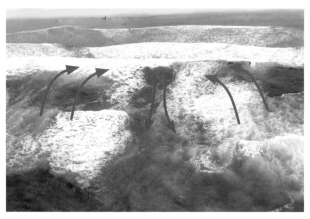

How to identify a rip

Inshore hole

An inshore hole is a trough that forms parallel to the shore; the depth may vary from a few centimetres to more than a metre. It is formed by the action of the sea, and unwary swimmers (particularly small children) can step into a hole or be swept into it by the backwash from a wave surge.

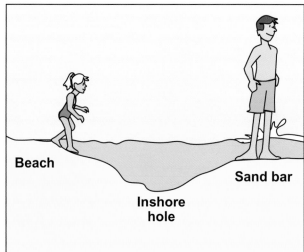

Inshore hole

Inshore drift currents

Inshore drift currents are side currents running parallel to the shore. A fast-flowing side current can sweep a swimmer along the beach into a rip current and out to sea.

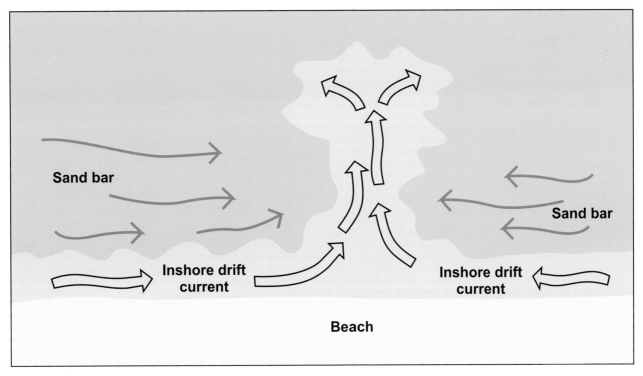

Inshore drift current

SAFETY TIP
If tangled in weeds, remain calm, remove weeds if possible, keep all movements to a minimum by trailing legs while using a restricted arm action to move out of the weeds.

Aquatic activities

Swimming is by far the most common aquatic activity, but fishing and boating are also popular and present their own inherent dangers.

SWIMMING

Swimming is a popular activity that can be enjoyed in swimming pools, at the beach, in the sea, rivers, lakes and dams. Unfortunately many incidents occur when people go swimming and are often a result of:

- not making an assessment of the environment before entering the water
- overestimating their own capabilities
- consuming alcohol, which affects their ability to make sound judgments
- not reading signs or obeying lifeguards.

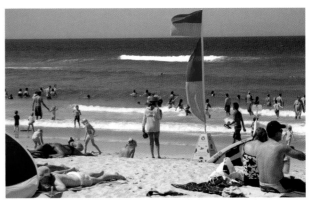

Swimming at the beach

FISHING

When going fishing, thorough preparation is required and suitable clothing and footwear is essential. People who fish from rocks should be physically fit and should possess competent survival swimming skills. The following precautions apply when fishing from the beach or rocks:

- check weather and tide details before departing and always ensure a safe passage to shore will remain when the tide begins to rise
- always fish in the company of at least one other person
- wear a personal flotation device (PFD)
- when wading across submerged reefs, be wary of obstacles and sudden drop-offs
- find a secure foothold when fishing from rocks
- avoid sloping and slippery rocks
- beware of being swept off rocks by a larger-than-usual wave
- avoid turning away from the sea
- do not mix fishing and drinking alcohol.

Fishing from a boat requires observation of the following essentials:

- check weather details before leaving
- always wear a PFD and carry required safety equipment
- always fish in the company of at least one other person
- do not mix fishing and drinking alcohol
- do not stand up in a boat to land a fish.

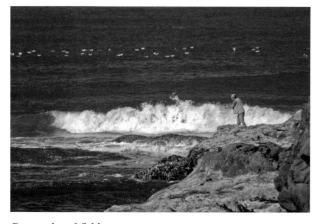

Recreational fishing

BOATING

Boating can be a dangerous activity unless safety precautions are observed. Boats should be inspected regularly to ensure seaworthiness. Equipment should be checked thoroughly to ensure it is present, in good repair, and conforming to government boating legislation.

The following guidelines should be observed:

- learn and follow the boating traffic rules
- leave word of the proposed destination and the estimated time of return
- check weather reports and monitor any deterioration in weather conditions, indicated by a build-up of clouds, wind rising quickly, or increasing swell and occasional whitecaps
- never take a boat out alone
- observe boat capacities to avoid overloading
- ensure that everyone on board wears a PFD
- carry all required safety and emergency equipment
- keep the weight centred and low when climbing aboard or ashore
- wear appropriate clothes and take extra clothing to allow for possible changes in the weather
- keep away from swimming areas, weirs, rocks and other craft
- learn and practise capsize and person-overboard drills
- if a boat cannot be righted in an emergency, remain with it.

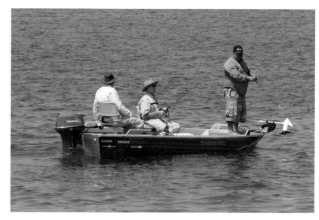

Boating — does this look safe?

DEPTH OF WATER

Extreme caution must be exercised when entering water when the depth is unknown. A dive entry in shallow water may result in a spinal cord injury. Diving entries should take place only in deep water in controlled swimming pool environments where the person has appropriate diving skills. Refer to Chapter 8 for more detail.

SAFE BEHAVIOUR IN AN AQUATIC ENVIRONMENT

- Never swim alone — aquatic activities should be undertaken in the company of others, preferably those skilled in rescue and resuscitation techniques.
- Use aquatic aids and equipment correctly — all items should be used in the manner they were designed for, with regular checks to ensure they are not faulty or damaged.
- Wear appropriate clothing — protective clothing for the weather conditions and activities should be worn at all times.
- Assess environment — before entering, assess the dangers, including depth of water, obstacles and currents.
- Know your personal aquatic capabilities — do not overestimate your ability or feel pressured to participate in activities you do not have the skills for.
- Abide by rules — safety rules, signage and lifeguards are there to alert the community to the dangers and inform the community about safe behaviour in an aquatic environment.
- Plan for emergencies — be prepared at all times.

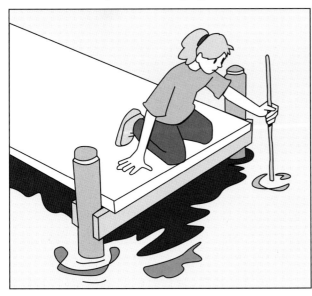

Always remember to check the depth of the water

TEACHING TIP

Reinforce to your students the importance of checking the depth of the water before entering.

SURVIVAL SKILLS

Students must have a realistic understanding of their personal abilities, the knowledge to assess the situation and form a workable plan of action, and the capability to perform survival skills.

Personal survival education should provide students with:

- knowledge of the specific dangers in each aquatic environment
- skill in applying a wide range of survival techniques
- the ability to select and perform the most suitable survival procedures
- the ability to improvise in the use of aids
- the capacity for endurance and skill in the water.

Entries

INTRODUCTION

There is a certain amount of risk involved in entering the water, particularly in unfamiliar aquatic environments. Selecting an appropriate entry into an aquatic environment is an important skill to learn to ensure that all safety factors have been taken into account. Firstly, carefully assess the environment in order to determine which entry may be the most suitable and also check you can exit safely. As safety is of utmost importance, the depth of the water, the clarity of the water, the possibility of submerged objects and the surrounding terrain must be considered. It is important to remember, particularly in open-water environments, conditions can change from day to day and an entry that was suitable one day may not be safe to use the next day. The following section outlines a range of water entry skills, when they are to be used and how to perform them.

Wade-in entry

When

- The water is initially shallow but the depth further out and conditions are unknown. This entry allows for the feet and an aid (if available) to feel for unseen obstacles and is controlled and safe.

How

- Ensure movement is controlled.
- Wade in slowly and carefully, keeping footwear on for protection, if possible.
- Slide the feet carefully along the bottom. If available, use a rescue aid (e.g. stick or pole) to test the depth, underwater obstructions and firmness of the bottom.

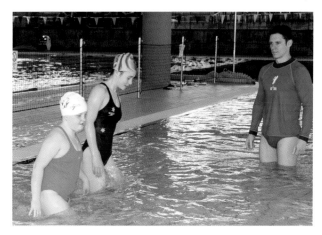

Wade-in entry

Slide-in entry

When

- The depth and the state of the bottom are unknown. This entry allows for the feet to feel for unseen obstacles and is controlled and safe.

How

- Ensure movement is controlled.
- Establish a firm body position, either sitting or lying with feet in the water.
- Feel with the feet for unseen obstacles.
- Lower the body gently into the water, taking weight on hands.
- Turn the head to the side with chin tucked in to protect the face from the edge during entry.

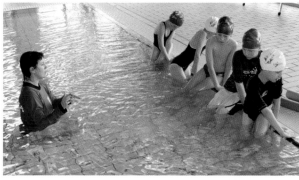

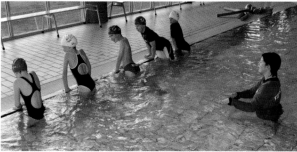

Slide-in entry

Stride-in entry

When

- When entering water known to be deep and free of obstacles from a low edge or bank. This entry allows a rescuer to keep watching a person in difficulty.

How

- Step out from a standing position, aiming for distance.
- Extend one leg forwards and the other backwards, slightly bent at the knees.
- Lean forward.
- Extend arms sideways and slightly forwards, elbows bent slightly and palms down.
- Look forward, to the person in difficulty.
- On entering the water, press down with the arms and scissor the legs to keep the head out of the water.

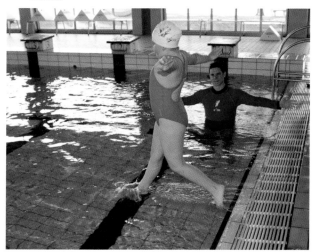

Stride-in entry

Compact jump

When

- When entry is from a height greater than 1 m into known deep water. This entry is mainly used in emergencies.

If not wearing a PFD

- Place both arms across the body with one hand over the mouth and nose.
- Step off with one foot leading.
- Bring legs together and keep them straight. Feet should be flexed, to 'punch' a hole in the water surface.
- Ensure body remains vertical, streamlined and protected with the arms across the body.
- Once under water, tuck the body to slow downward movement.

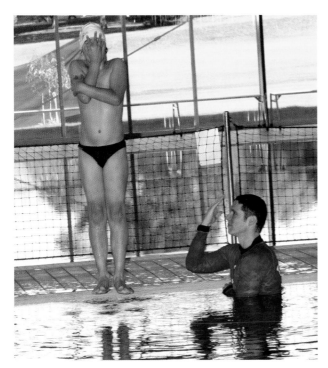

Compact jump (activity is performed in deep water)

If wearing a PFD

- Hold the PFD down securely to prevent injury to the head and neck when the device is forced up on entry.
- Jump feet first as explained above.

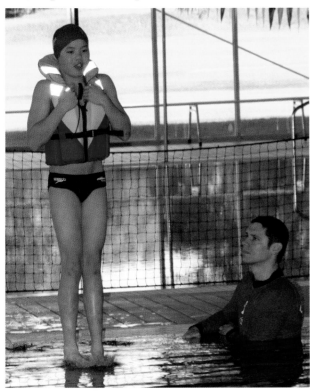

Compact jump with PFD (activity is performed in deep water)

Accidental fall in

When

- When a fall into the water occurs unexpectedly.

How

- Tuck chin onto chest.
- Hands placed on top of the head, protecting the face and chest with the forearms.
- Press elbows into the chest.
- Legs together with knees bent towards the chest.

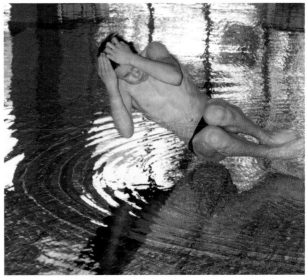

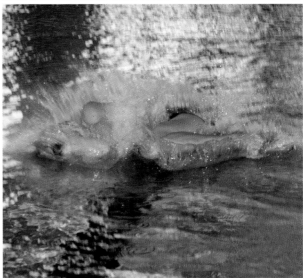

Accidental fall in

Dive

When

- The dive entry is used when the water is clear, free of obstacles and the depth is known to be suitable.

How

- Refer to Chapter 8, 'Teaching safer diving skills'.

> **SAFETY TIP**
> For more control and safety, curl toes over the edge when entering the water using any method. Always watch the area where you enter the water in case conditions change.

Exits

Leaving the water safely is an important survival skill. Wading, walking up steps and climbing ladders are considered natural, but exits that require physical strength, ingenuity or cooperation need to be learnt. Exits that simulate a variety of situations should be included in the program. For example:

- climbing into a boat
- climbing up a steep bank
- climbing up a muddy bank
- leaving the water with an injury
- climbing up a rope
- climbing onto a surfboard.

> **TEACHING TIP**
> Simulate a slippery/muddy bank by placing a number of PFDs along the edge of the pool and place a plastic sheet or foam over the top. Get your students to try and climb out, the wetter it is the harder it will be! Ensure this activity is conducted safely.

Signalling for help

The internationally recognised personal distress signal is one arm raised or waved above the head and a cry for help.

The best position for supporting the body while one arm is raised is the back float, sculling with one hand, legs kicking gently.

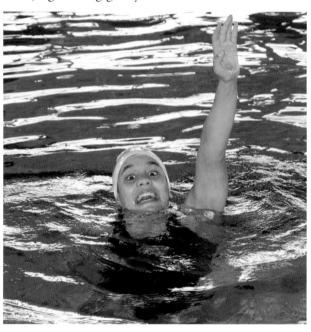

Signalling for help

Floating

Owing to body composition, some people find it difficult — or even impossible — to maintain a motionless float. However, floating is a valuable survival skill and may be possible for those who have difficulty with it if arm sculling and leg actions are used to give additional support. Floating is easier in salt water because it provides greater buoyancy than fresh water. The use of aids such as inflated clothing, a PFD, or a plastic container may assist flotation.

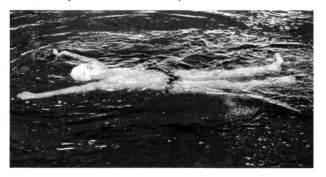

Floating

Sculling

Sculling is an important skill as it forms the basis of several other swimming and survival techniques. Sculling is performed by sweeping the hands outward and inward at a 45 degree angle, changing hand pitch at each change of direction. This action helps to produce uplift to support flotation. Refer to Chapter 7 for teaching techniques for sculling.

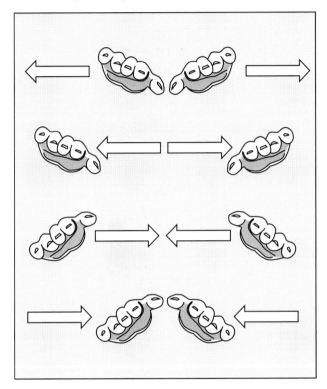

Sculling

Underwater skills

It is desirable to develop the ability to move about underwater with confidence. Swimming underwater and performing tasks, such as finding objects, tying and untying knots and removing clothing, are activities that can be practised.

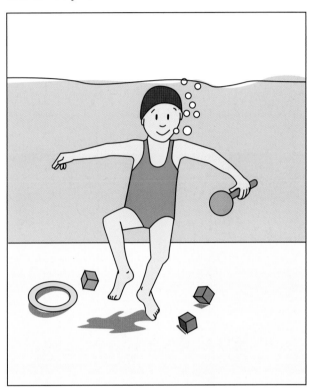

Underwater skills

Warning: Students must not be encouraged to take repeated deep breaths before swimming underwater or to hold their breath for substantial periods of time, as this can be extremely dangerous. This behaviour can lead to Hypoxic Blackout which is a severe reduction of oxygen to the body, which affects brain function leading to unconsciousness, and death, if a breath is not taken. If it occurs while in the water it can lead to drowning. It is recommended that activities such as underwater swimming competitions should be discouraged and not form a component of lessons.

Treading water and survival swimming

Treading water is a survival technique. It may be performed in either a horizontal or a vertical position. The horizontal position is preferred if the legs were to become entangled in kelp or water weeds.

Survival swimming involves using the most efficient energy-conserving technique possible. However, if a person is in a life-threatening predicament, such as in a burning boat, a speed stroke should be used to put distance between the threat and the person. For further information on how to teach treading water skills refer to Chapter 7.

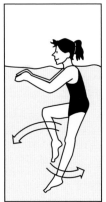 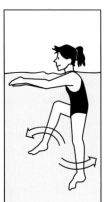 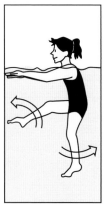 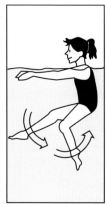 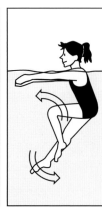 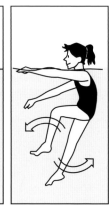

Treading water

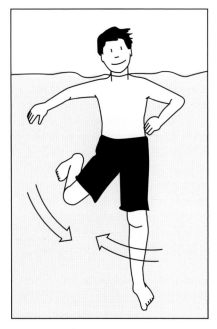 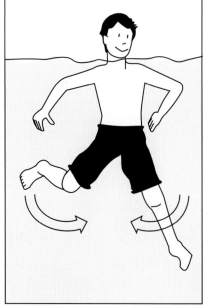 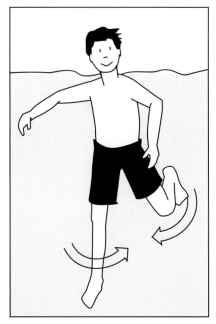

Eggbeater kick

Personal flotation devices (PFDs)

The use of various types of personal flotation devices (PFDs) should be experienced frequently throughout a swimming and water safety program. It is important to develop confidence in their use and to understand their performance attributes.

The PFD should be appropriately sized for the wearer. A small child may slip out of an oversized device and an undersized one will not provide adequate buoyant support for a large person.

> **TEACHING TIP**
> To ensure that students are competent in using PFDs correctly, a range of different skills should be experienced in lessons, including:
> – putting on a PFD on land and in water
> – using a PFD as a flotation support
> – getting in and out of the water wearing a PFD
> – throwing a PFD out to a person as a rescue aid.

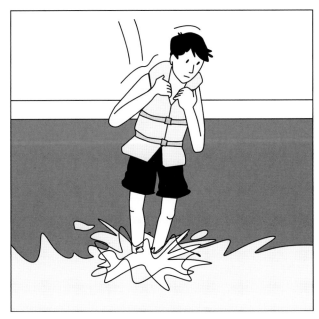

A personal flotation device (PFD)

Cold water and immersion hypothermia

Hypothermia occurs when the body core temperature falls (particularly of the heart, lungs and brain). Immersion hypothermia is an acute type of hypothermia produced when a person is immersed in cold water.

Normal body core temperature in a healthy person is about 36.9°C. This level is constant and is necessary for heart, lung and brain function. Maintaining the core temperature at this constant level is a function of a special section of the brain that is sensitive to small changes in deep core temperature. This section also monitors superficial temperature receptors.

Under normal conditions, the body copes well with exposure to cold or heat. However, when the difference in temperature between the cold environment and the normal body temperature is too great, heat loss exceeds heat production, the thermo-regulating mechanism fails and the body core cools. This normally occurs in water temperatures of 20°C and below.

When exposed to cold conditions the following symptoms may occur:
- intense and uncontrollable shivering
- performance of complex tasks is impaired
- difficulty in speaking
- shivering can decrease and be replaced by muscular rigidity
- thinking is less clear, general comprehension of the situation is dulled, possible amnesia
- unconsciousness
- most reflexes cease to function
- slow and weakening pulse
- in extreme cases, cardiac arrest.

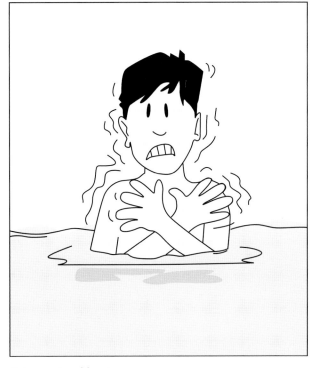

Exposure to cold water

WIND CHILL

It is important to understand the effect wind has on the temperature felt. The body cools itself by several methods, including radiation, respiration, evaporation, condensation and convection. The colder the air temperature the greater the heat loss from the body.

The body warms a thin layer of air around it and if this layer is blown away, a higher rate of heat loss occurs and the body feels colder.

COLD WATER SURVIVAL

A person who is unexpectedly immersed in cold water should not remove any clothing, except for a heavy item such as an overcoat, as clothing can help to prevent heat loss.

It is extremely difficult to judge distances in open water environments, particularly when rough and cold water can severely affect movement, coordination and stamina. It is only recommended to swim to a safer location if it is a short distance. If the person is close to the wreckage of a craft, they should attempt to climb onto the vessel, and maintain warmth by tucking into a ball.

Heat Escape Lessening Position (HELP) technique

A person wearing a flotation device can increase survival time by assuming the Heat Escape Lessening Position (HELP) technique. The knees are bent and drawn towards the chest, and the arms are pressed firmly against the sides of the chest. This position delays heat loss by protecting the most vulnerable areas: the head, the sides of the chest and the groin.

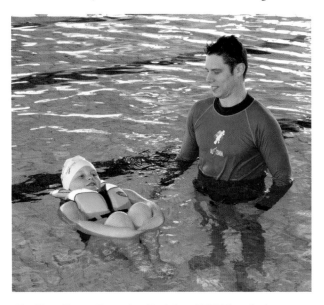

The Heat Escape Lessening Position (HELP) technique

Huddle technique

The 'huddle' technique is based on the same principle as the HELP technique and was developed for groups of three or more people. The sides of the chest, the groin and lower body are pressed together. This formation is particularly useful if small children are involved, as they can be supported, protected and warmed in the centre of the group.

If swimmers must stay in deep water without a flotation device for a long period, they should remain as still as possible, conserving energy and, if possible, in a tucked position. They should maintain this position through slow sculling of the hands. As the body core temperature drops it will become increasingly difficult for a person to make sensible decisions. Purposeful muscle movements (e.g. swimming or holding onto a boat) become difficult and people may be unaware of their situation.

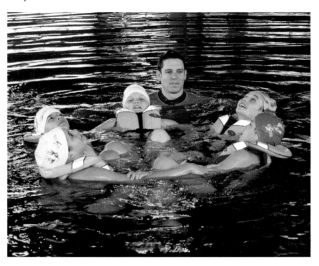

The huddle technique

Warmer conditions

HYPERTHERMIA

During the summer months people need to be aware of the warm conditions and the effects of strenuous, prolonged swimming in warm water.

It is easy to begin to experience hyperthermia and the associated effects of dehydration even when the weather is not extremely hot. Children are even more susceptible than adults to heat illness.

Steps to take to prevent heat illness include:

- avoid excessive activity during the hotter parts of the day
- drink cool water before, during and after activity
- wear cool, well-ventilated cotton-type clothing
- become acclimatised.

RESCUE SKILLS

Rescue principles

Most people learn swimming and water safety skills so that they can enjoy a wide variety of aquatic activities. As competence and skill increase, students progress to aquatic environments in which the margin of safety is reduced. It is vital that students gain an understanding of rescue principles and the lifesaving and rescue skills required to deal with an aquatic emergency.

Each emergency is different, and therefore the skills required to perform the required action will vary.

When assessing an emergency, students should consider:

- the degree of urgency
- availability of assistance
- the type of person in difficulty
- the distance from safety
- the weather and water conditions
- possible entry and exit places
- the availability of flotation aids or watercraft
- personal swimming and rescue ability
- the chances of reaching safety.

These considerations should provide sufficient information for an appropriate plan of action.

Recognising the person in difficulty

Many people still believe that a drowning person will splash and call for help. However, most are unable to signal for help, and they drown quickly and quietly.

There are four types of drowning victims, with characteristics peculiar to each, although in any case of drowning a combination of characteristics may be displayed. The characteristics of the four types of drowning victim are set out below.

The conscious non-swimmer:

- is in a vertical position
- is not necessarily facing the point of rescue
- is unable to turn around
- is unlikely to effectively use arms and legs for support
- is unlikely to respond to instructions
- is under water most of the time
- is unlikely to be looking for an aid to grasp; although may grasp the rescuer.

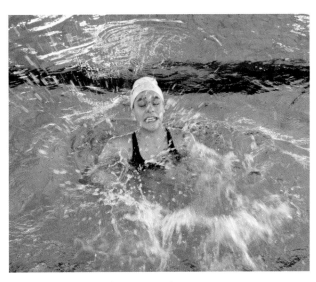
Recognising a conscious non-swimmer

The conscious weak swimmer:

- is in an inclined position in the water
- may use arms and legs for support
- may turn to face a point of rescue
- may wave or call for help
- may cooperate and obey instructions
- may grasp the rescuer.

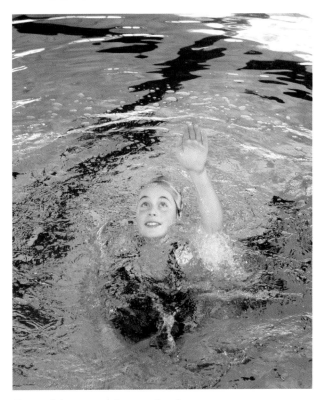
Recognising a conscious weak swimmer

The conscious injured swimmer:
- may be in an awkward position in the water and holding the injury
- may signal for help
- is concerned primarily with the injury
- may cooperate with the rescuer
- may have a spinal injury and be unable to move.

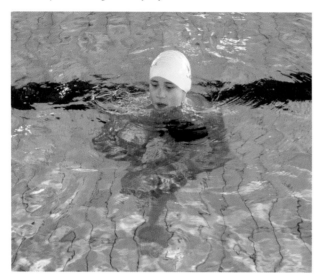

Recognising a conscious injured swimmer

The unconscious swimmer:
- is completely limp
- may be at any level in the water
- is often face down
- will offer no cooperation or response to instruction.

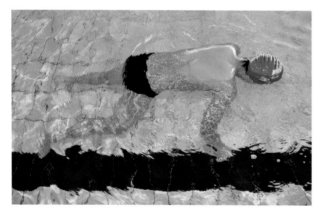

Recognising an unconscious swimmer

Self-preservation during rescue

The first and most important consideration for the rescuer in any aquatic emergency situation is self-preservation. If the person in difficulty grasps the rescuer, it is possible that both could drown.

FOR CONSCIOUS PEOPLE IN DIFFICULTY
If possible, the first attempt should be a dry rescue (talk, reach or throw).

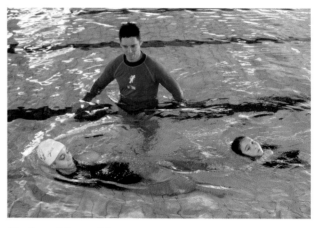

Towing with an aid

If the rescuer must enter the water, the following procedures should be observed.
- Always take a buoyant aid if one is available.
- If a buoyant aid is unavailable, take any aid that will keep a distance between the rescuer and the person in difficulty — T-shirt, towel, rope or pole.
- Approach the person in difficulty with extreme caution.
- Adopt a defensive position at a minimum distance of 2 metres from the person in difficulty.
- Reassure and instruct the person in difficulty.
- Encourage a non-swimmer or a weak swimmer to use the buoyant aid for support rather than providing contact support.
- Assist the person to safety, towing by the aid only when necessary.
- If an injured person needs contact support, note the location of the injury and take care not to aggravate the condition, particularly if it is a spinal injury.
- Only offer contact support if the injured person is cooperative.

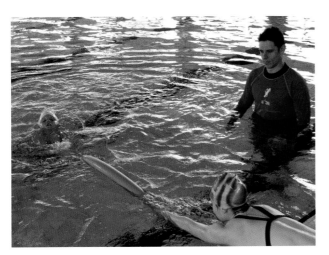

Attempt a dry rescue if possible

FOR UNCONSCIOUS PEOPLE

Observe the following sequence.

- Always take a buoyant aid if one is available, preferably one large enough to support the person.
- Approach quickly, remember DRABCD (danger, response, airway, breathing, circulation, defibrillation).
- Check for injury.
- Place the person in the most appropriate position (using the aid), with the airway open.
- Tow to safety as quickly as possible, supporting the person with the aid.
- Land the person — with assistance, if possible — and send for help.
- If there are no signs of life, continue with DRABCD.

If a person cannot be removed from water for any reason, then rescue breathing should commence in the water (rate: 15–20 breaths per minute). The casualty should be moved to dry land as quickly as possible, to enable commencement of CPR (cardiopulmonary resuscitation) immediately.

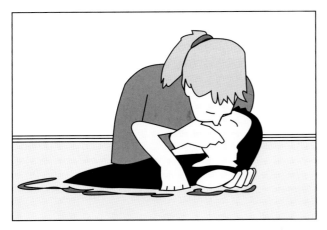

If a person cannot be removed from the water for any reason, commence rescue breathing

PLAN OF ACTION

If entry to the water is unavoidable, the rescuer's first action may be to obtain a flotation aid. Donning a personal flotation device (PFD) prior to entry may assist survival. Next, a safe method of entry must be selected. Once in the water, the rescuer must employ the skill most suitable in the prevailing conditions. However, conditions may change quickly so a person in a survival predicament may have to adapt both skills and plan of action quickly. When safety has been reached, the rescuer must make an evaluation concerning possible help from others, medical intervention and reporting of the incident to appropriate authorities.

Rescue techniques

THE RESCUER

To ensure the maximum degree of safety, rescue methods should be considered in the following order.

1. Talk
2. Reach
3. Throw
4. Wade
5. Row
6. Swim (with a rescue aid)
7. Tow

Methods of rescue should be selected and adapted to suit a rescuer's swimming ability, the condition of the person in difficulty and the rescue conditions. Each should be carefully studied to estimate the degree of risk involved. A rescue should never be attempted if the situation is dangerous to the rescuer and their personal safety could be jeopardised.

Non-swimming rescues should be the first method attempted and, where possible, entry into the water avoided. Whenever a swimming rescue is performed, the rescuer should approach with great caution and with the head up. A defensive position should be adopted to avoid being grasped by the person in difficulty. If the person lunges towards the rescuer, the rescuer should quickly reverse away.

The following section outlines when and how to use the rescue methods in priority order.

NON-SWIMMING RESCUES

Talk

Rescuing using your voice and signalling to assist the person in trouble is the safest form of rescue.

When

The person in trouble is conscious and capable of responding to instructions. They must be close enough to hear the rescuer's voice and to see the rescuer's gestures.

How

The rescuer talks and gestures to the person to encourage them to get themselves to safety.

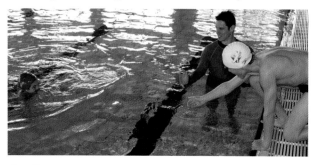

A talk rescue

Reach

A reach rescue should always be considered first in an emergency (if 'talk rescue' is not an option). It is considered both safe and effective for the rescuer.

When

The person in difficulty is near the edge. This rescue is suitable to perform for a weak or non-swimmer if necessary.

How

- Lie down with the chest to the ground.
- Keep the person under observation.
- Anchor firmly by using an assistant or fixed object.
- Reach out with an aid and instruct the person to hold it.
- Pull the person to safety slowly.
- If in danger of being pulled in, let go, then try again.

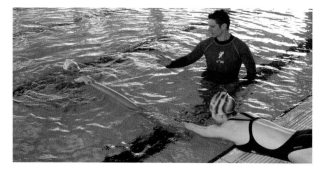

A reach rescue

Throw

A throw rescue can be used for weak or non-swimmers. A buoyant aid or a rope may be used.

When

The person is conscious but too far away to effect a reach rescue.

How

- Reassure.
- Choose a suitable aid. A buoyant aid or rope may be used.
- If choosing a buoyant aid (e.g. PFD) you must instruct the person to hold the aid to their chest and kick to the edge. Assist the person out of the water.
- If choosing a rope you must instruct the person to lie on their front or back and to hold the rope with both hands. If you are in danger of being pulled in, let go, then try again.
- If the person in difficulty does not respond or if the aid fails to reach the person, alternative techniques should be used.

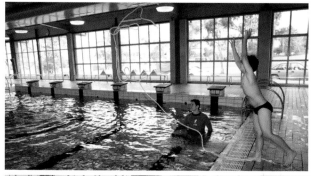

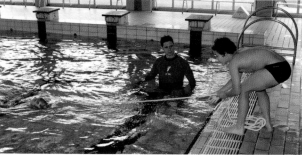

A throw rescue

TEACHING TIP

How to coil and throw a rope

- Coil the rope into even loops ensuring it doesn't tangle (with young children use full arm span to assist with getting even and large loops).
- Secure one end of the rope either with a foot on top of it or tying it to a fixed object.
- If the rope is long, split it into two even amounts with the end of the rope in the throwing hand. Make sure that the non-throwing hand is held out flat so the rope coils can run off when thrown.
- Throw the rope, aiming to land over the person's shoulder.
- Pull the person into safety, observing at all times, and secure them to the edge to assist in exiting.

Wade

When

To be used in shallow water when attempts to reach and throw have been unsuccessful or when the distance is too great.

How

- Reassure.
- Enter shallow water safely and if possible take a rescue aid (e.g. stick).
- Wade by sliding the feet along the bottom, testing the depth with the rescue aid.
- When the person is close enough, turn on your side and reach with the aid.
- When the person has grasped the aid, return to safety, but avoid any contact.
- If in danger, let go, then try again.

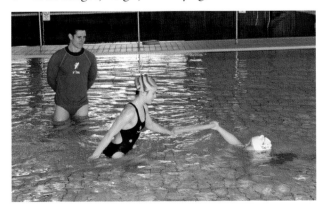

A wade rescue

Row

When

This is an effective and safe technique because the rescuer remains clear of the water and the person in difficulty can be secured safely and quickly.

How

Equipment such as a boat, wave ski or sailboard can be used, but the rescuer must be proficient in its use.

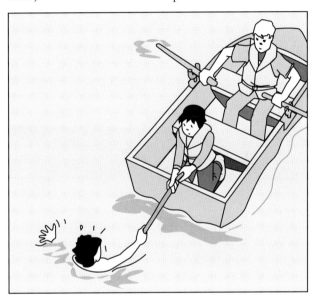

A row rescue

SWIMMING RESCUES

A swimming rescue should only be used when all land-based rescues have either failed or are not appropriate. Safety for the rescuer is of utmost priority and considerations for selecting suitable rescue aids, appropriate entry and landing, and approaching the person in difficulty must be made. It is essential for the rescuer to maintain a safe distance from a person in difficulty by adopting defensive positions. The first option for a swimming rescue would be an accompanied rescue but if this method is not possible or ineffective then a non-contact or contact tow should be used.

Swim

An accompanied rescue should be used when the person is conscious, cooperative and able to assist with the rescue and when a non-swimming rescue is not possible.

When

Should be used when the person in difficulty is too far from safety to be rescued by a reaching or throwing technique.

How

- Enter the water with a buoyant aid.
- Approach and reassure the person.
- Keep a safe distance.
- Adopt a defensive position.
- Pass the aid to the person and instruct them to grasp it firmly.
- Tell the person how to kick while holding the aid.
- Accompany the person to safety and provide reassurance throughout.

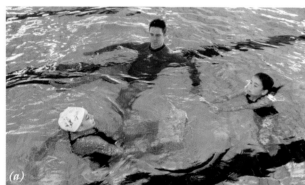

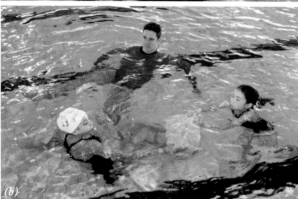

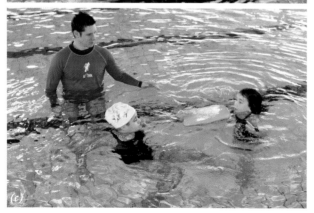

A swim rescue — (a) approach, (b) defensive, (c) pass aid

Tow

A tow rescue may be a non-contact rescue, when using an aid, or a contact rescue. A non-contact tow should be selected in the first instance if an aid is available, unless the person is unconscious. A range of contact tows may be used including cross chest, head, clothing, double armpit and wrist. The method of towing should be selected, taking into consideration the casualty and the environmental condition.

Non-contact tow

When

A non-contact tow can be used when an accompanied rescue is not possible or has been proven ineffective.

How

- Select a suitable towing aid, such as a rescue tube or ring.
- Enter the water safely and use a suitable approach technique.
- Adopt a defensive position.
- Inform the person what is going to be done, pass the aid and instruct the person to hold with two hands.
- Tow the person, maintain your distance, and keep observing.
- Reassure and encourage the person to assist by kicking.

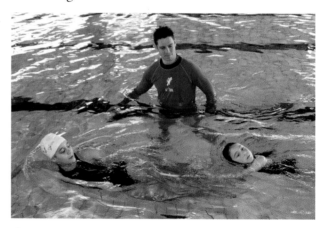

A non-contact tow

Contact tow

When

A contact tow is suitable for an unconscious person who is unable to assist. A contact tow for a conscious person who is extremely tired or severely injured may be used with extreme caution.

How

- If the person is unconscious, speed and safety is paramount.
- In the final approach, the rescuer should be cautious and defensive.
- Select a suitable towing method for the water conditions and type of casualty.

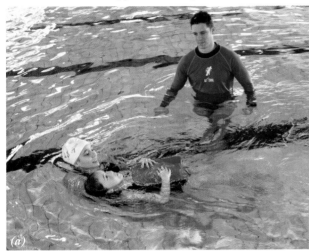

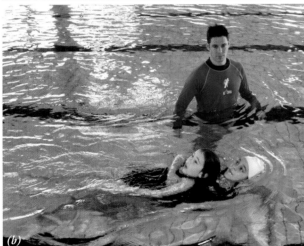

Contact tows — (a) with aid, (b) cross-chest tow

Defensive position

When

To be used when a rescuer approaches a person in difficulty.

How

- Maintain a safe distance from the person in difficulty.
- Tuck the legs rapidly under the body.
- Push the legs forward.
- Make a final assessment from this safe position.

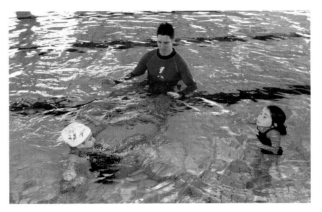

The defensive position

Reverse

When

To be used when the person in difficulty attempts to grasp the rescuer on approach or when the rescuer is in the defensive position.

How

- Tuck the legs rapidly under the body and push them forward, as in the defensive position.
- Kick away vigorously.
- Readopt the defensive position.

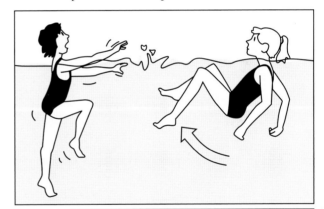

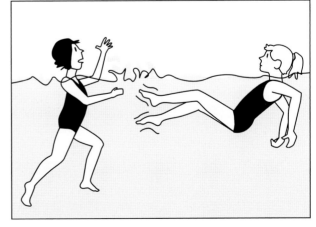

The reverse position

Assisted lift

When

To be used when the person in difficulty is unable to leave the water independently and additional help is available to assist the rescuer. When using this lift all assistants should adopt correct lifting techniques.

How

- One rescuer must take control and organise the lift.
- The person in difficulty should be facing the edge.
- The rescuers on the edge should take a firm hold of the person's wrists as the rescuers in the water prepare to lift each side of the person.
- On an agreed signal, all rescuers lift, raising the person to a position where the hips are level with the bank or pool side.
- Carefully bend the person at the waist, lower the trunk and head to the ground.
- Lift the person's legs out from the water, while turning the body to lie parallel with the edge, taking particular care of the person's head.

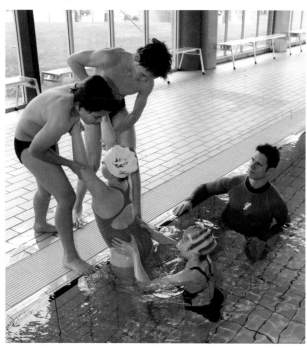

An assisted lift

CONDUCTING A SAFE AQUATIC PROGRAM

For information on how to conduct a safe aquatic program in an open-water environment refer to Chapter 10.

REVIEW QUESTIONS

1   Explain why water safety is important to include in all aquatic education programs.
2   List as many aquatic environments as you can and the potential hazards that may be involved with each.
3   List the different entry techniques you can use and explain when each should be used.
4   Explain these terms:
    - HELP
    - PFD
    - DRABCD.
5   List the rescue techniques you can use to help someone in difficulty. In order to ensure safety for the rescuer, arrange the techniques in order by which they should be considered.
6   Explain the following terms:
    - self-preservation
    - defensive position.

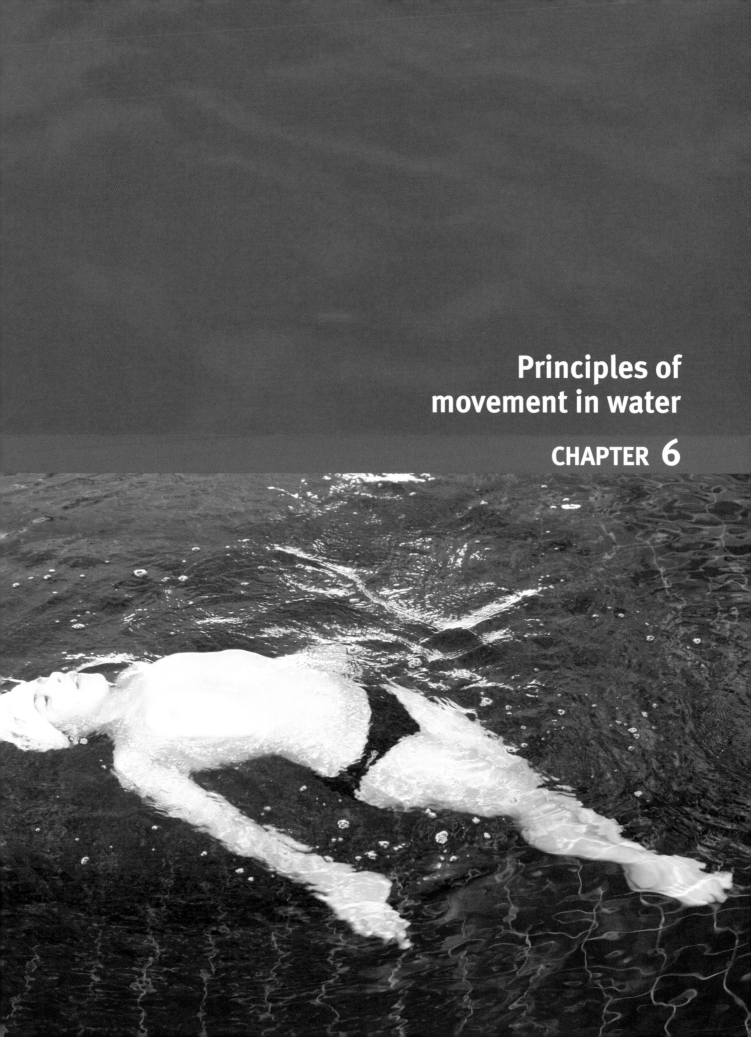

**Principles of
movement in water**

CHAPTER **6**

INTRODUCTION

Movement in and through water is affected by several natural forces. By understanding how these natural forces affect an object in the water, the teacher of swimming and water safety is able to teach movement patterns that best utilise these forces and is able to improve the quality of the students' performance. Knowledge of the governing principles of movement in water allows the teacher to provide correctional drills to help achieve efficient swimming techniques and better explain feelings and sensations. The teacher will also be better equipped to set achievable goals, taking into consideration individual differences.

Water offers a unique environment for humans. It possesses qualities that will assist the student but it also has qualities that will impede the students' progress through it. An understanding of the principles of movement in water and biomechanics (how the body moves) gives the teacher of swimming and water safety the basis to predict how water affects the body's movement. The actions of students in water depend upon the natural forces and their interaction with various internal forces generated by the student. Teachers with an insight into these forces and relationships and how they influence the body in water can utilise the positive aspects to maximise skill acquisition.

An understanding of how the body reacts in water assists in:

- improving performance
- correcting errors
- identifying ways to alter human movement patterns to improve stroke efficiency
- preventing injury
- building confidence.

As students gain a greater comprehension of the force of the water acting on and around them, they will become more proficient at using it to their advantage. The better use of the environment the student makes, the more efficient the student will be in moving through the water.

How efficiently the student moves through and uses the water will depend on the way their body interacts with the four forces on the body: gravity, buoyancy, propulsion and resistance.

- **Gravity** is the downward force of the Earth pulling on the body and cannot be changed or altered.
- **Buoyancy** is the upward force of water pushing on the body.
- **Propulsion** is the force that provides movement in the desired direction.
- **Resistance** is the force of the water which hinders movement.

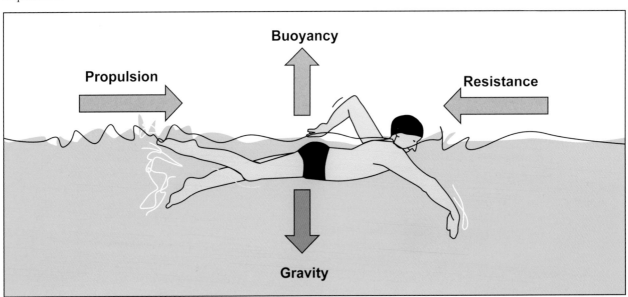

Forces affecting movement in water

BUOYANCY

The terms buoyancy and flotation are regularly used interchangeably and this is often not accurate. Flotation is one of the most important initial skills a student will be taught. It is the ability to maintain as much of the body on or near the surface of the water.

Flotation is achieved through the water pushing upwards on the body. This force is known as buoyant force. Buoyant force comes about because the body displaces (moves) water in order to be in it. Therefore, buoyancy is concerned with the force on the body and flotation relates to the student's ability to utilise that force.

Buoyant force

About 2300 years ago, Archimedes, a Greek scientist, observed that when he sat in his bath the water level rose and he felt lighter. From these initial observations Archimedes' principle was born. Archimedes' principle states that an object that is immersed in water (either partially or wholly) experiences an upward force as the water tries to stop the object from sinking. This buoyant force tends to counteract the effects of gravity and the weight of the object. This results in the weight of the object being reduced by the upward force of buoyancy. The amount of water displaced dictates the amount of buoyant force the body will experience. The bigger the body, the greater the amount of moved or displaced water and the greater the buoyant force upon it.

Students should be encouraged to experiment with buoyant force. This experimentation could take the form of submerging balls and balloons filled with air or trying to sit on the floor of the pool to experience the upward push of the water. Through experimentation students' understanding and confidence will increase.

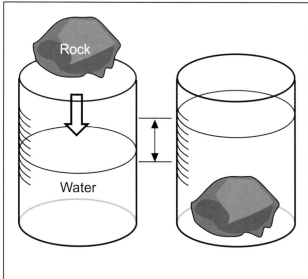

Buoyant force (see how the water level rises?)

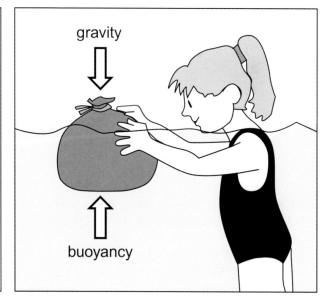

Density

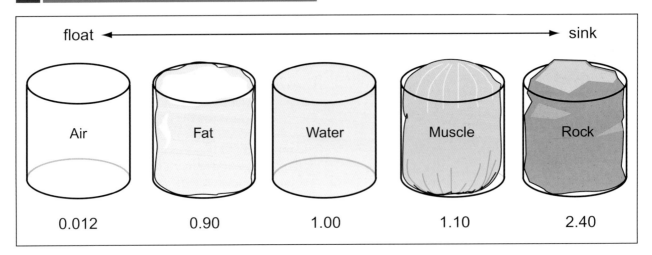

float ← → sink

| Air | Fat | Water | Muscle | Rock |
| 0.012 | 0.90 | 1.00 | 1.10 | 2.40 |

Explaining density

Density is the relationship between an object's mass and its volume. In swimming, water density is thought of primarily in terms of its affect on buoyancy. Water provides a buoyant force, but it also provides resistance to a student's propulsion. Of particular interest to teachers is the investigation of how the human body maximises the effect of naturally occurring forces of water.

The term 'specific density' refers to the difference between the density of an object and the density of pure water.

Pure water density is used as a reference point, having a specific density of 1.0. (This means that each litre of pure water has a mass of 1 kg.) Therefore, anything placed in water will float or sink according to its specific density value. Anything with a specific density greater than 1.0 will sink and anything less than 1.0 will float.

The density of the human body varies according to:
- the volume of air in the lungs
- the amount of fat in the body
- the degree of muscular development
- the bone density of the individual.

If the student's body contains a large amount of fat, which has relatively low specific density, approximately 0.9, then the body is more likely to float. However, a very muscular, lean body, or a body which has a high bone density is likely to sink. This occurs because both muscle and bone have a specific density of greater than 1.0.

In general, women float better than men because they have a higher percentage of body fat. Children generally float better than adults as their torso and lungs make up a greater percentage of their total body's mass.

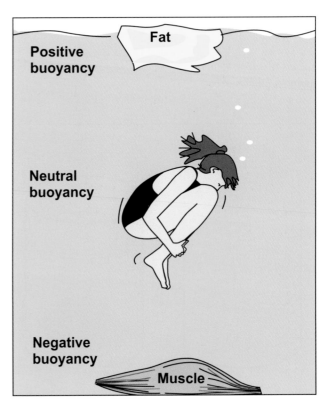

Positive buoyancy — Fat

Neutral buoyancy

Negative buoyancy — Muscle

Buoyancy and flotation

It is often said that we float better in salt water than in fresh water and this is correct. Salt water has a specific density of 1.03 and consequently will push up on the body with more force than fresh water.

Since individual differences will impact upon the student's ability to float, teachers need to be aware of the variation in density within each swimmer. Body shape, symmetry and breathing all affect the body's density.

Shape

The position of the limbs and head can drastically alter the floating position of the body. Small changes can alter the floating aspect in the water. Students should be encouraged to experiment with different shapes in the water and discover for themselves which shapes are most stable. Students should also be encouraged to float not only on their back and their front but also on their side and vertically.

> **TEACHING TIP**
> A novel way to enable students to experiment with shape and flotation is to get them to form as many letters as possible in the water (e.g. X, Y, I, O, L).

Symmetry and asymmetry

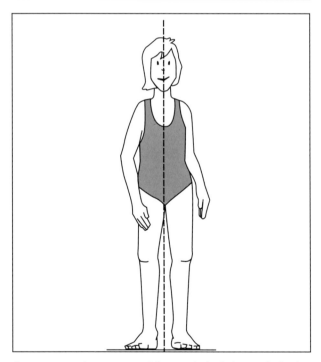

Symmetry and asymmetry (picture the body in two halves)

Symmetry and asymmetry will both impact upon a student in the water. A student who is symmetrical will have even distribution of mass and will be more stable when floating. A student, with an asymmetric body will not be evenly proportioned and will be less stable when floating.

Most human bodies have some form of asymmetry. For example, a keen tennis player will have greater muscular development in one arm than the other,

making that side of their body more dense. An older adult with a hip replacement will be asymmetric. Both cases will necessitate a change in body position to maintain a position of balance in the water.

The body's shape and symmetry will both impact upon the position a person will float in. Density will determine if the person floats or sinks.

Breathing

It is important that students realise that they need to keep breathing even when they are floating. While a large amount of air in the lungs may help a student to float, the student also needs to maintain their floating position in comfort. Encourage students to breathe normally when floating on their back and to exhale when floating with their face under the water.

Centre of gravity

Every object has an absolute centre position, and this is where the force of gravity acts upon it. This central point is known as the centre of gravity (CoG) and is the point around which the object balances. The CoG in a human is at approximately half the individual's height, as there is an equal spread of mass above and below this point. As a practical method of finding your own CoG, imagine you are a see-saw, your CoG is the point about which neither your feet nor your head touch the ground.

Centre of buoyancy

The centre of buoyancy (CoB) is similar in position to the CoG but slightly closer to the head, as above and below this point there is an even spread of displaced water. It is often easier to think of this as the mid-point of buoyant matter (e.g. fat and air). To demonstrate this in the water the teacher can use a plastic ruler and two pieces of plasticine. By changing the position of the pieces of plasticine the ruler will float in different positions, the same way people do, depending on how the fat and air is distributed in their body.

Floating horizontally

Every object that is immersed in water is subjected to an upward force through the CoB and a downward force through the CoG. These two opposing forces, acting through different locations in the body, produce rotating forces. These rotating forces result

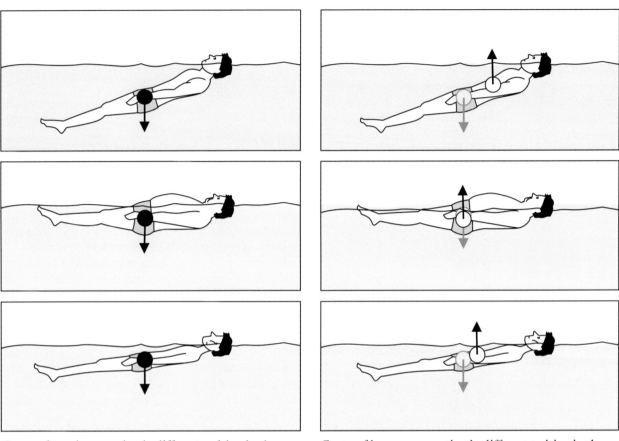

Centre of gravity — notice the different position in the water for each body shape

Centre of buoyancy — notice the different position in the water for each body shape

in a rotation of the body. In order to float horizontally the CoG and CoB need to align vertically through the mid-section of the body. It is very difficult to shift a student's CoB, however it is possible to manipulate their CoG to bring it in line with the CoB. Changes in the shape of the student's body that shift the weight

towards the head result in the CoG moving in the same direction. Moving the hands above the head, bending the knees and lifting the fingers slightly out of the water all help in moving the CoG towards the head. This movement assists the body to attain a horizontal, motionless floating position as the CoG

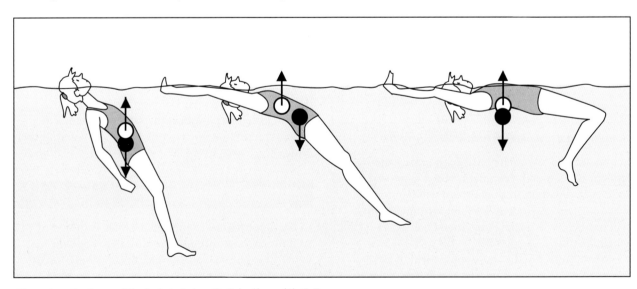

Changing the shape of the body to bring CoG in line with CoB

and CoB become aligned. Many people are unsure about how sticking the fingers out of the water helps with horizontal floating and this is because the fingers (out of the water) are heavier than if they are under the water. While the fingers are in the water they are affected by gravity and buoyancy, however if they are out of the water then they are only affected by gravity.

A person who floats easily is likely to learn swimming and water safety more readily than one who has difficulty in floating. However, an individual's progress should not be restrained because of an inability to maintain a motionless float; in many cases this will never be possible. Any movement or rotation that occurs during floating will therefore be the result of the CoG and CoB being out of alignment. Factors that may cause this to occur include shape and symmetry (as mentioned above).

For many students it is difficult to maintain a horizontal float and for a small proportion it is impossible. These students have a greater density than water. While most children and women have a density of less than 1.0 and float, there are some people whose density is greater than 1.0 and, therefore, they sink. In order for a student who sinks to float they will need to move and create a propulsive force which lifts them to the surface. One of the simplest propulsive forces is lift force and this is described later. A student who sinks while performing a stroke or drill is failing to produce enough lift force to keep them afloat.

This is usually the result of poor sculling technique and an inefficient kick. Good underwater arm and hand actions will ensure sinking does not occur.

> **TEACHING TIP**
> The position of the head largely determines the position of the body in the water. The body acts in much the same way as a see-saw; if one end is up, the other is down.

Rotation

Rotation occurs when the CoG and the CoB are trying to align themselves vertically. Rotation can be destabilising during floating but can be controlled and used for recovering from a floating position (see Chapter 7 about floating and movement).

VERTICAL ROTATION

Generally, a student's legs will sink lower than the upper body as they are denser than the water they have displaced. The position at which the body will come to rest and float in the water is found when the CoG aligns with the centre of buoyancy. When this occurs the CoG and the CoB will be acting as directly opposing forces. This type of rotation is known as *vertical rotation* and can be summarised as movement forwards or backwards.

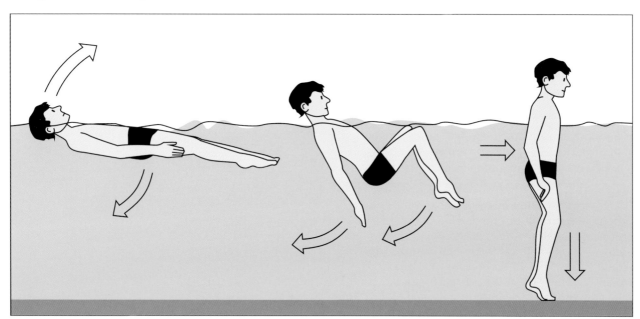

Vertical rotation

LATERAL ROTATION

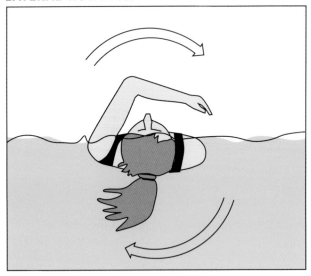

Lateral rotation in the horizontal plane

Lateral rotation occurs from side to side. The body often rotates quickly as the axis it is rotating around is short and is offered very little resistance from the water. This type of rotation can be controlled by changing the body shape. An easy change is to make the axis of rotation longer by stretching one arm out from the body.

PROPULSION

Propulsion is the positive qualities of the water that students use to move in a desired direction, whether that direction is up, forwards, backwards or sideways. It is generally accepted that in a stroke such as freestyle the hands and arms provide at least 80% of the propulsive forces; in some swimmers they are the only source of propulsion.

> Both the arm/hand and legs/feet propel the body through the water, with the arm/hand responsible for the majority of the propulsion.

To obtain a better understanding of the body's propulsive forces, close examination of the hand and arm action under the water is necessary. Try this for yourself — stand up and 'swim' through the air. How far did you go? Nowhere, because your hand has trouble grabbing the air to pull you forward. This time grab the end of a bench or table and 'swim'. Your body is pulled, propelled, forward. Why? A swimmer's body will only move forward if the hand or foot is applying a force to a relatively stationary surface. It may feel as though the foot goes backwards in breaststroke and the hand goes backwards in freestyle

and butterfly, but this is really not the case. It is the body that moves forward and away from where the propulsive forces are generated (representing action and reaction). The hand of the swimmer can be compared to the foot of a runner. If the runner cannot apply force to the road, then their body will not move; therefore if a swimmer cannot grip the water then they too will not go anywhere. So, when swimming, our body actually moves past our hand, our hand doesn't move past our body. Of course this is not strictly accurate, a highly efficient swimmer can grip the water more efficiently to pull themselves through the water, a novice's hand will slip a little in an effort to catch the water.

Thus forward movement of the body occurs when a force is applied to a surface that remains stable. The objective of the swimmer is to apply force to the water with the hand, without allowing the hand to travel backwards through it. The magnitude of the force needs to be great enough to overcome the water's resistance and the weight of the body in the water.

There are two forces that enable the student to move forward in the water:

1   Lift force — creates an area of low pressure on the back of the hand which sucks the swimmer towards the direction the back of the hand is facing.
2   Water friction — uses the water's frictional forces to push against.

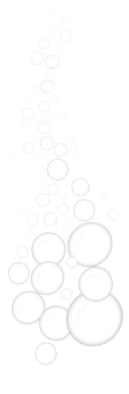

Lift force

Lift force is created when the hand moves sideways through the water. The sideways movement decreases the resistance on the hand and at the same time creates lift as the water flows smoothly across the hand's surface. The principle of lift force (also known as Bernoulli's principle) is the same principle by which aeroplanes fly.

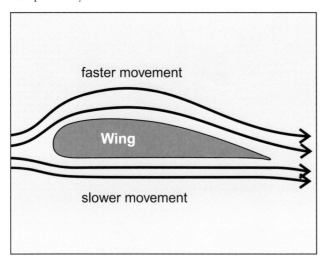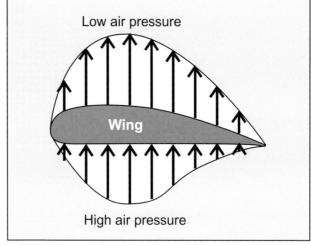

Lift force on an aeroplane

As the back of the hand has a greater surface area than the front, the water moving across it will move faster than the water moving across the palm. This creates a difference in the speed of the water travelling on the back and palm of the hand. This difference in speed/velocity creates a difference in water pressure around the hand. The faster moving water on the back of the hand creates an area of low pressure, and the slower moving water on the palm of the hand creates an area of high pressure. The high pressure pushes into the low pressure and, because it is between the two pressure systems, the hand is pushed towards the low pressure.

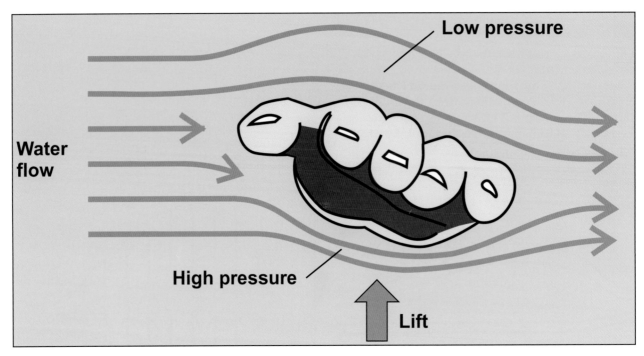

Lift force

TEACHING TIP
Sculling is an elementary propulsive skill and will assist the beginner to float and move.

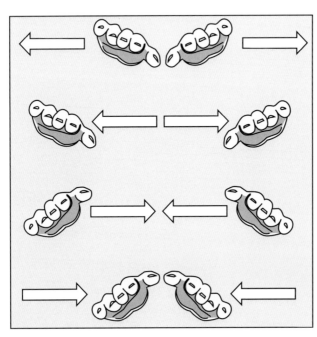

Sculling action

Lift force is most commonly used when sculling.

As the hand moves sideways constantly there is a continuous pulling of the body towards the low pressure on the back of the swimmer's hand. By changing the pitch of the hand the student can change their direction of travel. For example, a swimmer who is on their back with their fingers tilted towards the surface will move head-first. Whereas the same swimmer with their fingers tilted towards the floor will move feet-first.

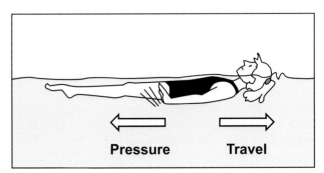

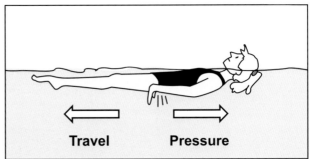

Changing the pitch of the hands will change the direction of travel

When teaching sculling; try to encourage students to obtain a 'feel' of the water. In order to enhance this sensation get them to push and pull the water, wearing socks or stockings on their hands.

> **TEACHING TIP**
> Try to use a catch phrase such as 'thumbs up and in, down and out' to illustrate the motion of the hand in the water.

Sculling and lift force are used in all strokes. For example, the catch phase of freestyle and backstroke utilises the principles of lift force — as the hand enters the water, it moves sideways, catching or gripping the water. This sideways movement is a half scull. Lift force and sculling highlight the need for good hand position through the water and good hand entry position.

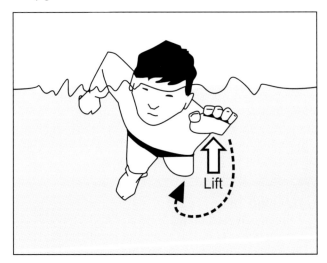

Swimming stroke demonstrating sculling and lift force

> **TEACHING TIP**
> The back of the hand usually faces the direction of travel and therefore dictates hand entry and catch positioning.

Water friction — action and reaction

As a swimmer applies force against the water with the hand a slight pressure is experienced; this is the result of the water rubbing against the surface of the hand as the water tries to slide past the hand's surface. The frictional resistance of the water provides a base for the hand to push upon, and the body is able to move forward via the principle of action and reaction. This means that if the hand pushes down on the water then the reaction is for the body to move up in the water.

This pairing of action and reaction is the cause of many common errors in the beginner student. For example, beginner students often travel from side to side, in a zigzag manner. Any sideways movement is a result of the body trying to balance itself. This occurs because the arm enters the water across the midline of the body and the legs try to compensate to balance the body. This creates a zigzag or snaking action, where each alternate arm entry causes the legs to move in the opposite direction. For each alternate arm entry, the legs move wide and cause a zigzag. The student can overcome this by developing an efficient hand and arm entry, and a strong, effective kick.

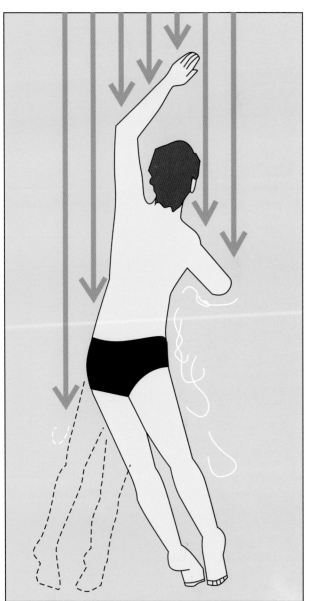

Effect of excessive side-to-side body movements

Bobbing, particularly in freestyle, is another problem many beginner students demonstrate. This occurs because the student attempts to go faster by pushing down on the water. The reaction to this action is that the body bounces or bobs up in the water. A smooth rhythmical arm action and a still head will assist the student, but changing the pitch of the hand and arm so that they push backwards and not down will have the most effect in correcting the beginner.

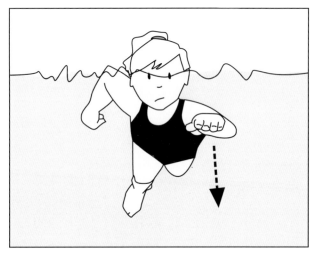

The body 'bobs' up and down when pushing directly down on the water.

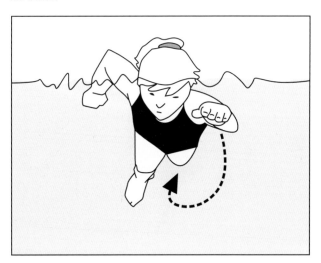

Prevent 'bobbing' by altering the pitch of the hands and arms

Levers

A crowbar or an oar on a boat are good examples of levers. The human arm and leg are built-in levers, without which we could not walk or pick things up. Within the human arm there are three sub-levers, fingertip to wrist, wrist to elbow and elbow to shoulder. It is often easy to think of the arm as an oar. If the arm moves as one lever, from shoulder to fingertips, then the pivot point (called the fulcrum) is located in the fingertips. The amount of force that can be applied to operate the lever is related to the size and strength of the muscles in the shoulder joint alone. This is the same as rowing a boat — the amount of force that can be applied relates to how hard you can pull/push on the end of the oar.

This means that the amount of force we can apply to an arm lever is limited by the strength in the shoulder muscles. However, if the arm is broken into its three sub-levers and bent slightly, this engages the muscles at the end of all three levers; wrist, elbow and shoulder. There are now more muscles involved in levering the body through the water. This enables the student to apply more force to their levers and they will swim more efficiently, because they are utilising more muscles. Bending the arm not only makes the student swim 'faster' but also decreases the likelihood of shoulder injury as less pressure (force) is being put on the shoulder joint and muscles alone.

TEACHING TIP
An ineffective action places much stress on the shoulder joint. It is therefore important to encourage students to bend their arm slightly during the propulsive phases of the strokes.

RESISTANCE

Resistance occurs because the water is not inclined to move out of the way when we move through it. It resists in three ways: skin, frontal and eddy resistance.

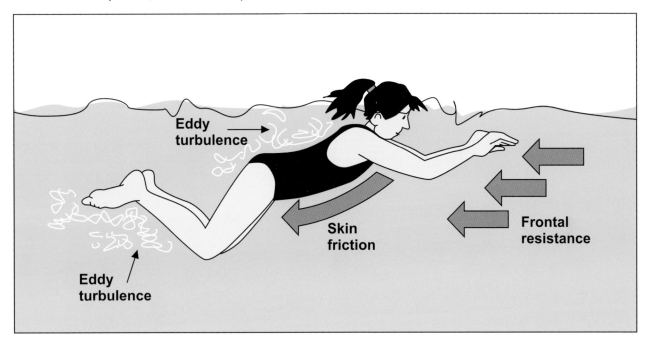

Three forces of resistance

Skin resistance

Skin resistance, or friction, is the friction that occurs between the skin of the body and the water. This form of resistance occurs because 'new' water is always rubbing against the swimmer's body. If neither the skin nor the water are moving then there is no friction and therefore no resistance.

The magnitude of the skin resistance is determined by:

- the speed of the water relative to the speed of the student — the faster the student or water is moving the greater the resistance
- the surface area of the body — the more surface area a student has the more friction will occur between it and the water
- the smoothness of the body surface — a rough surface rubs more and creates more friction and this is why many elite swimmers shave their bodies before competition as it makes their skin smoother and consequently less resistant.

Skin resistance can be reduced by wearing close-fitting swimming costumes, shaving, and wearing swimming caps. The teacher and the student have very little control over the amount of skin in contact with the water.

Frontal resistance

As the student moves forward in the water, the smooth flow of the water is interrupted by their shape and position in the water. The interruption in flow slows the progress of the student. Frontal resistance can be thought of as the water pushing against the 'front' of the student (front being the widest width and depth of the student's body which pushes through the water). Frontal resistance depends on factors such as:

- the size and shape of the student — the bigger the front moving through the water the greater the resistance
- the body position of the student — the more streamlined a student's body position is, the less resistance
- the speed of the student — the faster the student is trying to move through the water the greater the frontal resistance
- the student's technique — the more efficient the swimming technique is, the less frontal resistance.

Frontal resistance is most easily reduced by decreasing the size of the front moving through the water. The student's body position becomes very important in decreasing frontal resistance; a long narrow body position will decrease frontal resistance. A practical example to use with beginners is that of a sleek sports car and a large truck.

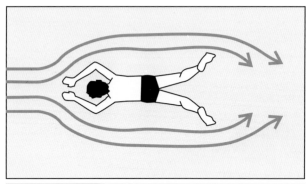

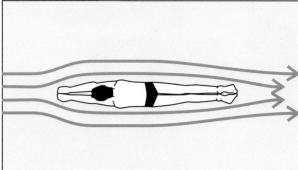

Demonstration of frontal resistance

TEACHING TIP
It is important to ensure that students acquire a streamlined body position during the early stages of stroke development.

As mentioned previously, poor technique also plays a major role in increasing frontal resistance. Examples of poor technique often exhibited by the beginner include students whose bottom sinks during backstroke, therefore increasing the front that needs to pass through the water, and breaststroke with wide knees. Both of these faults can be corrected by improving the student's body position and decreasing frontal resistance.

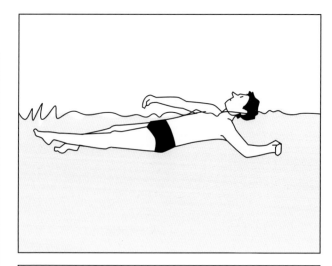

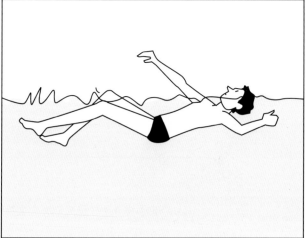

Poor technique will increase frontal resistance

To demonstrate the effects of frontal resistance to students, get them to push off the wall in the shape of the letter I (streamlined) and observe how far they travel. Get the students to repeat the action but this time in the shape of a T. Students will see and feel how important the streamlined body position is in going further and faster with less effort.

TEACHING TIP
The legs and feet tend to be used to stabilise the body in water and keep it streamlined.

Eddy

As the human body is an irregular shape it causes the water to be disturbed as the student moves through it. The disturbed water 'tumbles' in behind the body, creating eddies of swirling water. The water swirls because it is rushing around the body to fill the space previously filled by the swimmer. This vacated area is an area of low pressure which 'sucks' everything near it into itself, including other water and the body. The strength of the eddy will depend on:

- the size and shape of the body. The bigger the body, the greater the eddy resistance.
- the smoothness of the body surface. The smoothness referred to here is different to the smoothness referred to in skin resistance. Here smoothness relates to the sharpness of the body; for example, a circle as compared to a square.
- The faster the water flowing around the swimmer the greater the eddy resistance.

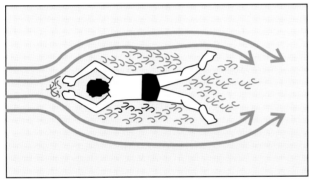

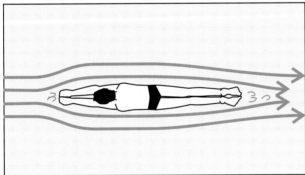

Water swirling in an eddy

In order to minimise the effects of eddy resistance a streamlined body position is important as it reduces the irregularity in the student's body shape.

Eddy resistance is not all bad; it is used often to assist the beginner learning to swim, and for the more experienced student to increase efficiency. For example, a student floating in front of their teacher who slowly moves backwards will create an eddy between themselves and the student causing the student to be sucked towards the teacher. Slipstreaming is an example of experienced swimmers, cyclists and car drivers using the eddy created by the person or object in front of them to 'suck' them along. However, eddies can cause a beginner swimmer to move backwards. When students try to perform a drill or complete a stroke, sometimes they do not travel forward efficiently and appear to move backwards or stay stationary. This reflects the student's inability to effectively catch the water and propel themselves forward. Excessive turbulence is often created by the dragging of air bubbles under the water. When eddies form around the body, the suction created prevents the body from moving forward. A good streamlined position plus effective arm and leg actions will prevent backward movement.

REVIEW QUESTIONS

1. Explain what buoyancy is.
2. What is the Archimedes' principle?
3. What are the factors that affect the density of the human body?
4. Explain the following terms:
    - centre of gravity (CoG)
    - centre of buoyancy (CoB).
5. What is lift force, and how does it affect a swimming stroke?
6. Explain the types of resistance against the body when it moves through the water. Provide examples of how you can work towards reducing resistance.

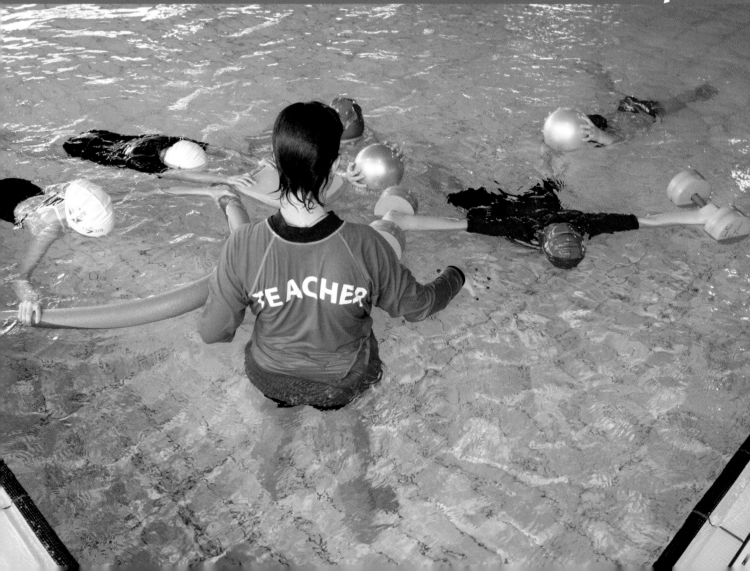

Water familiarisation, buoyancy, mobility and safety

CHAPTER 7

The swimming and water safety program aims to:
- encourage the development of a student's confidence in the water by providing a wide variety of activities in safe environments
- increase students' awareness and understanding of the need for water safety by teaching the appropriate knowledge, skills and activities
- encourage the development of swimming strokes and water skills which form the basis of recreational swimming and aquatic activities
- encourage the development of personal water safety skills.

INTRODUCING A STUDENT TO THE AQUATIC ENVIRONMENT

Ideally, the first contact that students have with the water should be an active, enjoyable, fun experience. Carefully graduated progressions which reinforce positive experiences should be developed by teachers of swimming and water safety.

The initial stages cannot be rushed. Students must be able to progress at their own pace and according to their own abilities. They should be given time to explore what their bodies can and cannot do.

It is essential that teachers understand the needs and fears of each student. Teachers should offer reassurance and encouragement, and sense when students are apprehensive about a particular activity. If students are reticent to attempt something new, teachers should recognise the need to take a step back and reintroduce the activity via another approach.

Students constantly challenge their teachers. For the teachers, this stage can provide one of the most rewarding times in teaching swimming and water safety. Few things can rival the satisfaction of observing reticent students develop into 'water happy' people, eager for their next lesson.

Force has no place in the teaching of swimming and water safety. Force can instil fear and produce negative results, often to the stage where beginners do not want to participate. Positive feedback is the best method of reinforcing the development of skills. Praise works wonders in forming good habits and motivating students. Students must have confidence in their ability to attempt an activity.

A teacher's success can be measured by the confidence and overall happiness of their students.

Trust is a vital element, for without trust there is fear and little enjoyment; without enjoyment, there will be little practice and, without practice, students will not consolidate the skills or develop the positive attitudes required to learn.

Fun activities and games are essential in learning. Students, young or old, will achieve more through enjoyment than fear. Through enjoyable games and activities, skills can be introduced without students even realising; their attention is more on the activity than on their possible fear of the water.

The knowledge and foundation skills students must acquire before further skills are introduced include:
- water familiarisation
- buoyancy and flotation
- mobility.

Learning through these stages is critical prior to the introduction of stroke development.

The importance of being confident and competent in water familiarisation, buoyancy and mobility skills cannot be underestimated. Movement through these skill stages is like a chain, with each link closely connected to the others. Progression through these stages should be with encouragement, praise and understanding from the teachers.

As the students develop confidence in the water and develop trust in their teacher, activities in deeper water can be introduced. Taken slowly and with lots of encouragement, teachers can help students to become accustomed to deeper water.

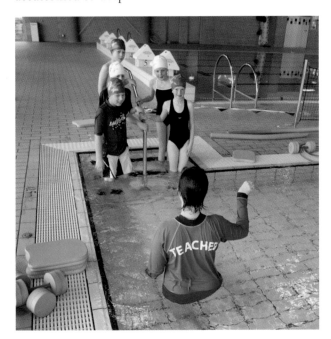

Introducing a student to the aquatic environment

Student needs

Students need teachers who have good skills and who are friendly and consistent. Other factors that are important for students are:

- comfortable water temperature
- clear, clean water
- familiar surroundings (e.g. location of deep water, toilets, entry and exit points)
- knowledge and understanding of the safety regulations
- defined class areas
- a friendly class atmosphere
- success within the lesson
- working with others of similar ability
- direction in the correct use of flotation aids
- class areas that are free of distractions
- 'dry activities' areas for out-of-water activities (e.g. cold days).

For students, becoming familiar with water is a whole new environmental experience. Teachers should not expect students to arrive for the lesson knowing and understanding complex sets of aquatic movement/ motion principles. Students, on entering the water, experience first-hand how their body is affected by water.

STUDENTS DISCOVER FOR THEMSELVES THAT IN WATER:

- walking requires more effort
- falling over is like falling in 'slow motion'
- it is more difficult to regain their balance when they fall over
- they experience a feeling of heaviness around the chest and a restriction in breathing when they wade into deeper water
- they experience sensations of semi-weightlessness.

Students must not only become familiar with the water and their new surroundings, but also with other children and adults who are initially strangers to them. They may feel very anxious about entering the water, but equally concerned about being left with teachers who are unknown to them. Teachers must understand these concerns and exercise care and patience in helping beginners to adjust to this new environment.

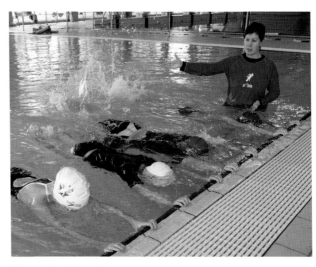

The student's needs

WATER FAMILIARISATION

Simply stated, familiarisation relates to the time, activities and support we all require to become comfortable, relaxed and familiar with something. In our case it is water and the aquatic environment.

If the familiarisation stage is too rushed we remain apprehensive and unable to learn. If the familiarisation stage is too slow we become bored and disinterested, and again, unable to learn. Getting the balance right is an ongoing challenge for teachers, because familiarisation is an ongoing process that will occur every time something new is introduced. It's this challenge that makes the teacher's role so interesting — no two days and no two students are ever the same.

The first step in teaching is familiarisation, and there are several critical factors that relate to the human body in water that must be understood and considered by AUSTSWIM teachers before the familiarisation process can begin. These include:

1 body position and density
2 vertical and lateral rotation
3 balance
4 extremes of body position.

1. Body position and density

Alterations in body position and density will impact on all people in water to varying degrees. A student may be affected by an alteration in body position or in density or a combination of both.

It is possible to predict the effect of changes in body position on a person's balance in water.

It is vital that teachers look at the student's body position, as this enables advice and instruction to be given on what action to take to maintain good balance and control in water. This will enhance the student's comfort and degree of control in the aquatic environment.

The severity or alteration of a student's body position will dictate the amount of control the student has over the degree of roll and the angle the body will float.

FACTORS IMPACTING ON BODY POSITION

- tenseness
- shutting the eyes
- holding the breath
- involuntary movement such as:
  - shivering
  - nervous jerking or shaking.

DENSITY

The weight, height and build of a person's body will determine how their body will react when immersed in water.

Understanding body position and density will enable the teacher to explain what is happening to the student's body and how to counteract body rolling in order to maintain a position of stability.

2. Vertical and lateral rotation

There are two forms of rotation (rolling) in water — vertical and lateral. Head movement is the influencing factor of the human body in water. Head movement will greatly impact on a student's ability to master and control both vertical and lateral rotation. For example, as a student moves their head backward (by looking up to the roof or sky) they may find themselves suddenly floating on their back. Likewise, by moving the head forward the student may find themselves in a face-down float position. These rolling actions often result in students finding themselves in a situation where they are unable to recover to a safe standing position, consequently they may panic or become distressed.

VERTICAL ROTATION

Vertical rotation is the forward and backward movement of the body that impacts on the student's ability to recover to a safe standing position from a front or back float. Vertical rotation includes moving from a standing to lying position and vice versa. Recovery from a lying to standing position involves bringing the knees up, reaching forward with the hands, pushing the head forward and breathing out.

LATERAL ROTATION

With this side-to-side movement of the body in water, lateral rotation occurs quickly as the human body offers little resistance and even less control for the beginner.

When standing, lateral rotation is turning the body left and right. When lying in water, lateral rotation rolls the body left and right. In this position the student is very unstable and must be taught to achieve control of rolling movements as lateral rotation is the most common cause of fear and anxiety in the water. Mastering control of lateral rotations is essential for confident balance in water.

Few human beings have a completely symmetrical body shape; this increases lateral rotation and can be counteracted by altering the position of the body in water. Moving or altering the position of an arm, leg or the head will assist in gaining control of lateral rotations.

> **TEACHING TIP**
> It is vital to teach understanding and control of rotations. Changing body position by repositioning the head, arms or legs will impact on rotation of the body.

Head control is of vital importance and must be taught in all activities. For example, a beginner standing in water whose face is splashed will react by moving the head back sharply, and probably sideways, to avoid the splash. This action of the head will cause an immediate forward and upward movement of the feet, with an associated rolling action of the body. The result will be a student who has no control over their body and who cannot recover to a safe standing position.

3. Balance

The ability to balance the body in any position against water turbulence (movement) is essential. Students must learn to stabilise their positions when faced with a loss of balance. Students should be given opportunities to achieve balance in the following positions:

- standing
- sitting
- kneeling
- lying (floating back and front)
- full rotation (rollover) from front to back floating
- somersault
- combination and movement from one position to another.

4. Extremes of body position

There are two extremes of position when the body is in water ranging from streamlined to extremely non-streamlined.

Of the two extremes, the 'streamlined' posture is what we are ultimately aiming for as it is very efficient in water. However, gradual steps must be taken to ensure a student's comfort and confidence. Gradual progress is vital during the following stages:

- water familiarisation
- buoyancy
- mobility
- safety.

STREAMLINED BODY POSITION

In a standing position the body is vertical, feet together, arms by the side. The body is taking up a very small area and may be easily disturbed or fall forward, backward or sideways with little or no turbulence present.

For stability, students should be encouraged to stand in water with head slightly forward, arms and feet out wide, in a slightly crouched position to maintain sound balance.

When floating in water the streamlined body position is very unstable for the beginner as the body will roll from side to side (lateral rotation).

The impact of the streamlined body position is most evident when a student is learning to float. Many teachers use a kickboard to introduce this skill, instructing the student to 'hug' the kickboard to their chest, lie on their back and float. This is extremely unstable, creating the side-to-side (lateral roll) and an immense amount of tension in the student who may panic when trying to recover to a safe standing position.

Using two flotation aids, or a noodle, will enable the student to create a wider more stable body shape, thus reducing the effect of the side-to-side (lateral) roll.

NON-STREAMLINED BODY POSITION

Balance is more stable when the student creates a wide body position that is in a slightly curled position. As balance and control develops the body position can be 'unrolled' and limbs moved closer to the body to create a longer, more streamlined position.

Adjustment and readiness

Before a student can begin to learn the art of horizontal movement in water, they must first start with the foundation basics of water familiarisation. Outlined in Table 7.1 are some steps that should be used as an introductory guide to ensure students are stable, confident and ready to move onto the next stage of learning and development.

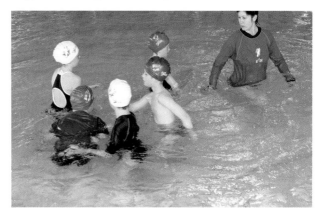

Adjustment and readiness — foundation basics

Simple progression

The temptation to quickly move a student from a vertical to horizontal position is enormous. After all, 'swimming' is achieved only in the 'horizontal' position. Parents, your peers and supervisors, indeed the students themselves, all want to see traditional horizontal 'swimming', however, vertical balance and stability must first be achieved.

Movement from vertical to horizontal should be progressive, moving from the crouched wide/ball-type shape, to a banana-type shape and finally 'unrolling' to a more streamlined position (see Table 7.2).

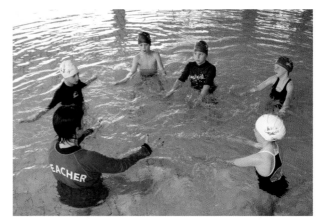

Adjustment and readiness — simple progressions

Table 7.1 Adjustment and readiness	
Apprehension	Students may be unsure of what the lesson consists of, or what will be expected of them. Time must be allowed for a comfort zone to be reached.
Fear of falling	The lack of something 'solid' to grasp contributes to this feeling. This fear is real and needs to be acknowledged. Mastering rotations and recoveries will help overcome this fear.
Inability to move as easily as on land	Rapid quick movements and reactions happen easily on land with little thought involved. Movement in water is slower and requires more effort. Often a student will become frustrated with this slow movement, and some students may fear they cannot 'get back up' for a breath quickly enough.
Spatial and body awareness	The judgment of distance, distortion of body position, the movement and expanse of the water, can result in a problem with spatial awareness. Working within small, well-defined areas and including regular body pattern work will assist a student to understand where body parts are in the water and how to use them effectively.
Breath control	A rhythmic breathing pattern should not be assumed; it should be taught. Each person must be capable of taking in a breath and be able to blow it out when the face is in, near or under the water.
Water has weight	Students must understand that water can be leant against, pushed against and used to enable movement and propulsion. On land the air around us 'parts' easily, allowing us to move freely. However, immersing the body in water requires us to exert more effort and energy to 'move' or 'part' the water to enable us to be mobile.
Land movements	Since birth the human body learns a myriad of skills that eventually enable vertical movement (rolling, sitting, crawling, walking, running, jumping, hopping, skipping and so on). The ability to maintain stability, balance and confidence against water turbulence, while standing, walking, turning, sitting and lying in water are essential to successful aquatic education. Re-learning these 'land-based' skills in an aquatic environment is an essential step for the beginner. Complete comfort and stability in water must be achieved in a vertical position before progressing to a horizontal position. Balance through movement is an essential foundation skill for the beginner.
Feel of the water	The sensation of water upon the skin and the drag effect behind the body moving through water must be experienced.
Deep-water drift	Immersion in water also creates movement of water. This will impact on the beginner, creating a drift toward deeper water. Teachers of swimming and water safety must be aware of this and be vigilant in supervising each student's ability to overcome and counteract the drift towards deeper water.
Temperature	Other than being in the bath at home, students may have little or no experience of immersion in water. Teachers need to be aware that inactive students will be very prone to feeling cold. This will increase body tension and reduce the student's comfort.
Aquatic readiness	Activities should be performed with increasing independence; ensuring progress is suited to the individual student.

Table 7.2 Simple progressions	
Leg movement	A simple kick action can be introduced and will be a very inefficient bent leg or even a cycling motion. Progression through the water will be minimal, however, distance is not the aim; comfort, balance and stability are the prime focuses. As confidence builds, the student can be introduced to a more traditional leg action.
Arm movement	Large arm movements, especially those that require above-water recovery, should be avoided for the beginner. Moving any limb out of the water creates instability and will result in lateral rotation. Simple hand-sculling action is recommended and can progress to greater movement of the arm and hand. It is beneficial for the beginner student to practise hand and arm/hand-sculling movements in a standing position, experiencing the different 'feel' of the water at varying degrees of hand immersion. Progression continues with arm movements in a horizontal body position. Again propulsion and distance are not the primary focus; comfort, balance and stability are the aims. As confidence increases the student can be encouraged to adopt a small above-water hand recovery. This can be done as either dual recovery or opposite hand recovery. Simple progression can continue to a more traditional swimming arm action.
Combined movement	When comfort, balance and stability are achieved, together with a confident recovery to a safe standing position, the beginner student should be encouraged to combine a simple kicking action with a sculling action. Simple progression can continue to more traditional swimming action.

TEACHING TIP
Propulsion and distance are not the primary focus. Students should be given opportunities to practise skills over short distances with many repetitions to ensure maintenance of stability and control.

BUOYANCY AND MOBILITY

Now that students are familiar with the water and have 're-learnt' their land skills (standing, walking, running, jumping) in an aquatic environment, we can begin the introduction stages of buoyancy and mobility.

The aim at this stage is for students to:
- experience weightlessness and buoyancy
- become confident in their ability to float independently in different positions
- learn to control buoyancy and body rotation
- be able to return to a safe, stable standing position.

Many people have difficulty in achieving a motionless float because of the high proportion of muscle and bone in the body, and may have to use sculling actions to maintain surface buoyancy. In these cases it will be necessary to combine buoyancy and mobility activities.

Students at this stage need to learn to raise their feet off the bottom of the pool, become fully supported by the water and then return to a safe, stable standing position. To accomplish this, they need activities that will help them to discover and understand the buoyancy characteristics of water. The following experiences should be included:
- floating on their front, back and side on the surface of the water
- floating in a variety of body shapes: stick, ball, banana
- quick bob-down attempt to sit on bottom (in shallow water) to feel the 'upthrust' sensation
- using the limbs to maintain a horizontal float
- using the limbs to maintain a vertical float
- using the limbs to maintain an underwater position
- breathing activities
- water safety activities with and without a variety of flotation aids.

TEACHING TIP
During the teaching of the buoyancy stage, teachers may need to call on skills from the water familiarisation and mobility stages to help students relax and grow in confidence.

Lesson plans during the teaching of the buoyancy stage should include:
- new, enjoyable activities to introduce mobility to students
- activities that reinforce water familiarisation skills
- buoyancy skills practice.

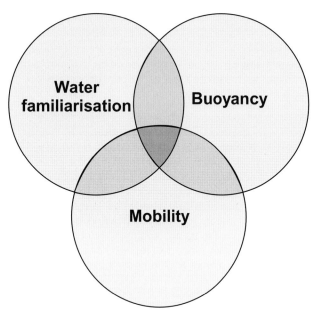

The total swimming program

Surface buoyancy on the front, back and side

FLOATING ON THE FRONT

Teachers should introduce floating on the front by floating in shallower water or by using a platform.

A variety of methods can be used including:

- using a pool wall, ledge or side
- using noodles
- using two kickboards
- use 'muscle bars' or pull buoys.

Students hold onto the side, edge, or flotation aids with feet on the bottom. The torso is extended and the chin is on the surface. A full breath is taken, the face placed in the water and held there while the teacher counts slowly to three. To exaggerate the effect of buoyancy, students should exhale slowly while under the water, and thus feel the body sink further as more weight is placed on the feet.

The head should then be raised slowly to just clear the mouth from the water and the previous action repeated. The teacher could ask students what is holding the body up or whether they are able to feel the rise and fall of the body, and the reason for this.

From the same starting position, students can take a deep breath, hold it fully, extend the body and try to wash the back of the head or look for the navel while placing the face in the water.

Many students will find that the feet naturally float to the surface and that the body will not sink. Others may need to be encouraged or even directed to allow the feet to float upwards.

> **TEACHING TIP**
> When first learning to return to a standing position (recovery) from a floating position, directions should be given regarding tucking of both knees, lifting the head and pushing down with the hands to assist with the action. Many students need to practise and be assisted with this process to avoid a loss of confidence.

The process must be continually repeated until the students have achieved reasonable success in floating with their faces in the water. A further stage could be to repeat the activity, but when the feet have floated up to the surface, allow one hand to gently let go of the edge, ledge or flotation aid and float free.

Learning to float face downwards

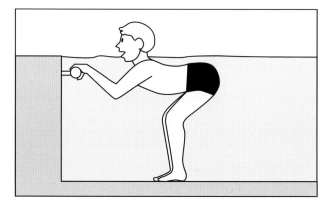

Take a breath, step 1

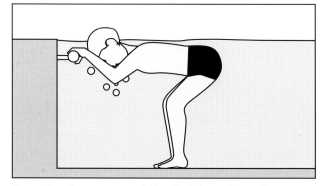

Lower face into water and blow bubbles as feet walk backwards and arms extend, step 2

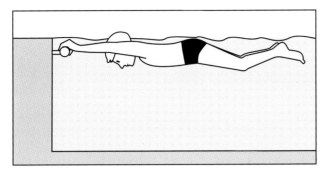

Floating face down, step 3

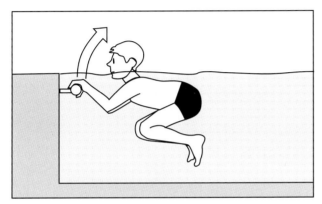

Draw knees to chest with head out last, step 4

Progressions for front float

- One hand grasps the wrist of the hand holding the wall/floatation aid. This hand is released when the feet float.

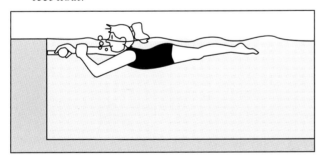

Progressions for front float, step 1

- The above is repeated, but with both hands letting go of the wall/flotation aids and pressing down in the standing-up stage. (Sometimes students are more confident working with a partner for this exercise.)

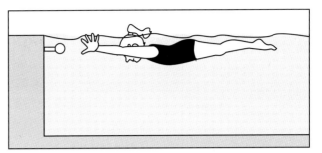

Progressions for front float, step 2

- One person stands in front of another who assumes the floating position. The support partner does not let the floating partner drift away.

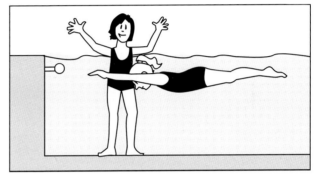

Progressions for front float, step 3

- The person takes a small step away from the wall and reaches forwards to float into the wall, but remains in a float position, holding the wall for a count of three. This can be repeated, with the person being progressively moved further from the wall.

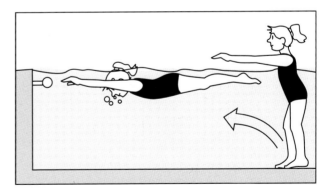

Progressions for front float, step 4

- Encourage students to open their eyes (looking for objects, fish or the wall). For those who are less confident, the teacher may place a hand under the water for them to watch or reach towards.

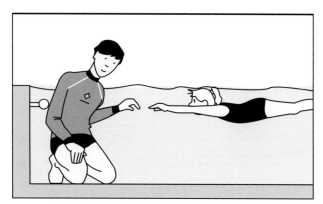

Progressions for front float, step 5

- Standing up before reaching the wall should then be introduced. Then, facing away from the wall, students can float or glide to a designated target.

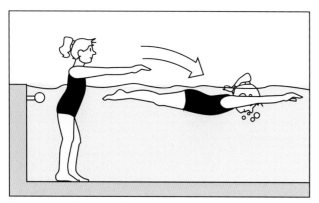

Progressions for front float, step 6

Practising in shallow water

- From a kneeling position, with the hands apart on the bottom, students place the face in the water, straighten one leg at a time, and allow it to float up to the surface.

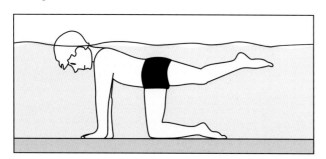

- With the chin in the water, students take a full breath, place the face down in the water and allow the legs to float up to a relaxed (wide) position. They then ease air slowly out of the mouth.
  With the chin alternately in the water and on the surface, they walk the hands along the bottom like a crocodile, expelling the air noisily.

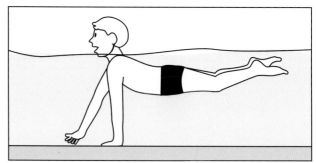

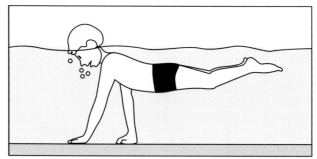

- Students place the face in the water with both hands on the bottom and, as the feet float up, allow one hand to float up gently. They then stand by pressing down with the floating hand, pulling the knees up and raising the head.

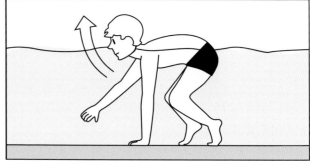

Learning to float face downwards in shallow water

EXPERIENCE AND EXPERIMENTATION

Experiment with a variety of flotation aids, floating on the back with recovery to a safe standing position.

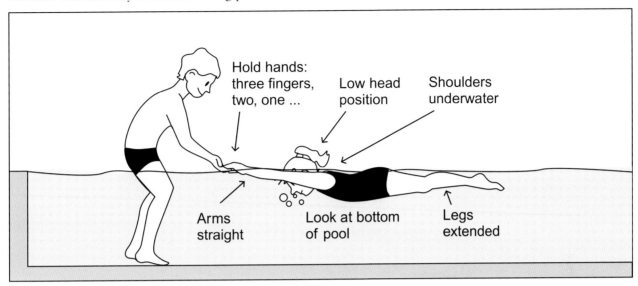

Front float using partner for support

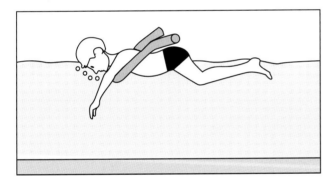

Front float using flotation device

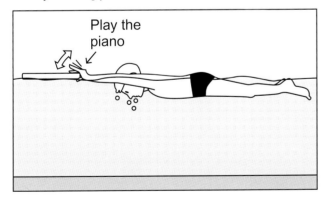

Front float using flotation device and piano technique

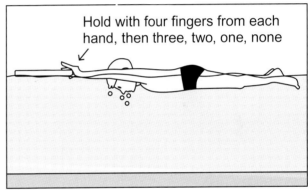

Front float using flotation device and progressive finger removal

TEACHING TIP

For sound body orientation and floating, try further variations using a variety of different body shapes, as this will not only assist with body orientation, but will greatly enhance adjustment to the aquatic environment.

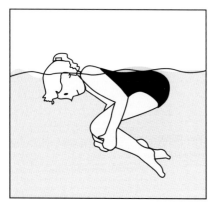

Body orientation and flotation variations — mushroom float

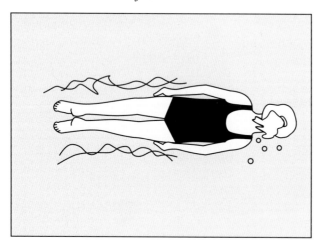

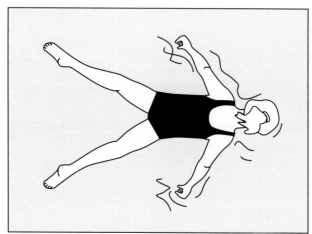

Body orientation and flotation variations — star float

FLOATING ON THE BACK

Floating on the back can be learnt progressively. If available, the initial practice can be undertaken in very shallow water, where the students can experience lying down in water. It is often a new sensation to feel water in the ears and 'hear' the sounds of water.

> **TEACHING TIP**
> Wide body shape, stability and control are key factors to back-floating success.

Try these activities

Using a buoyant aid, such as a noodle around the waist or two kickboards under the armpits, ask students to slowly lean back, lower the back of the head onto the noodle and extend the hips while looking up. To recover to a stable position, students raise the head, bring knees toward the torso (sitting position) and place feet on the bottom.

Students sit in the pool with the hands resting behind the hips and lean backwards until the elbows rest on the bottom. From this elbow-rest position, the upper body leans back until the shoulders and back of the head submerge and the top of the forehead is level with the surface of the water. From this position, the hips are pushed towards the surface with the eyes looking up at the sky. This is repeated and then the arms straightened until fingertips provide the only support.

To stand up (recovery), students tuck the chin into the chest, pull the knees upwards as the hips sink, push down with the hands and extend the legs to stand.

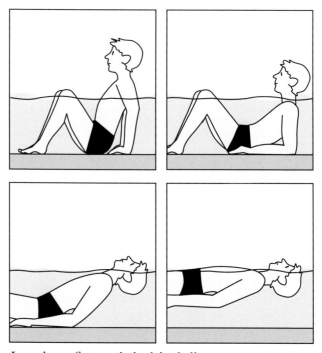

Learning to float on the back in shallow water

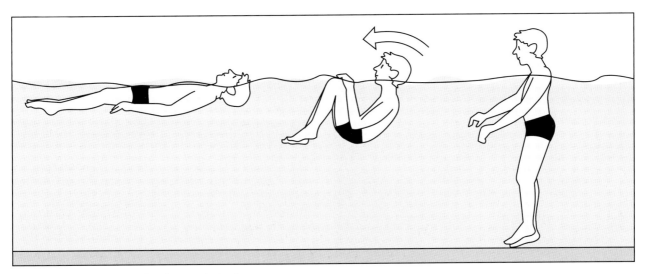

Regaining balance from floating on the back

Side floats

Many of the shallow-water activities mentioned in the front and back float sections can be used to teach the side float:

- using the elbow for support
- with a flotation aid held over the hips or held out past the head.

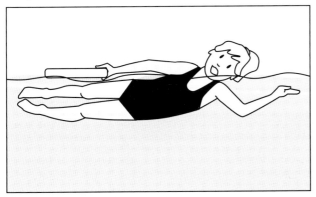

Side float

Using the limbs to maintain an underwater position

Students should be provided with an opportunity to explore the various limb actions required to maintain an underwater position. The following activities should only be carried out in clear water:

- shallow water:
  - lying on back or front on the bottom of the pool
- waist- or chest-deep water:
  - various body positions (front, back, curled, wide etc.)
  - various depths (midway, bottom, surface).

Students can perform these activities while remembering to practise exhaling (fast and slow for variety).

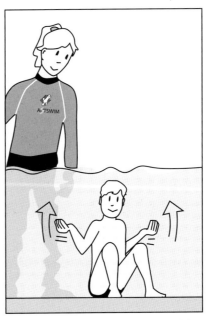

Maintain an underwater body position

Experimenting with buoyancy

Students can experiment with buoyancy using a variety of flotation aids:

- buckets
- water mats
- water logs/noodles
- other flotation aids.

The following activities will enable students to discover that various flotation aids have different degrees of buoyancy:

- floating in different positions using various flotation aids
- floating with an aid and then kicking to the edge
- group floating.

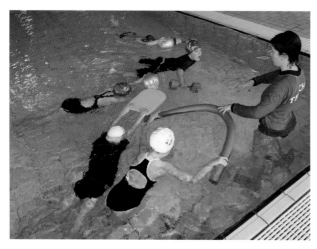

Experimenting with buoyancy — on front

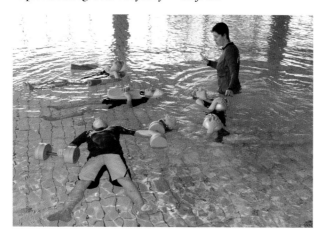

Experimenting with buoyancy — on back

CHANGING FROM ONE FLOTATION POSITION TO ANOTHER

The development of confidence and sound body orientation skills must include student's experimenting with fluid movements that change from one float position to another.

Students should be encouraged to move slowly, keep the limbs in the water, feel for positions which are easiest to maintain and move the limbs to maintain a balanced, buoyant position. Students can try:

- mushroom float (holding/hugging legs)
- jellyfish float (this is like a mushroom float, but the arms and legs are dangling like tentacles)
- turtle float (this is like a mushroom float, but the head is lifted to get another breath of air without standing, the head is then placed back in the water)

- floating like different letters of the alphabet or shapes.
- star float (front/back)

Students should experience these floats in various combinations (e.g. star float on front, changing to a mushroom and twisting over to a back float).

Breathing activities

Breathing activities should constantly be reinforced with all practices and will give students the experience of exhaling underwater. (Refer to page 99.) These activities can be done both with or without assistance from the teacher.

MOVEMENT THROUGH THE WATER (MOBILITY)

Once students are familiar with the water and have good orientation, body balance and buoyancy skills, it is time to introduce movement or basic mobility and propulsion.

The aim of this section is to:

- enable teachers to give students the opportunity to discover and explore limb movements that will propel them through the water in different body directions (head first, feet first and sideways)
- help students understand the principles of propulsion through the water, especially the effects of body position and streamlining.

The activities used should allow students to explore ways of using the arms, the legs or both the arms and legs to move on the surface or underwater.

A paired action

A paired action occurs when both the arms or both the legs perform a similar action (e.g. streamlining, the breaststroke action or the butterfly leg kick).

An underwater recovery

An underwater arm recovery occurs in strokes when the arms don't break the surface of the water. The arms are returned to a position under the water to begin the propulsion phase of the stroke (e.g. the breaststroke and survival backstroke arm actions).

An alternate action

An alternate action occurs when the propulsion phase of a stroke is being performed by one arm and/or leg, while the other arm or leg is performing the recovery phase (e.g. the freestyle arm action).

An above-water arm recovery

An above-water recovery occurs when the arm is lifted out of the water as it returns to the entry position (e.g. the freestyle arm action).

An independent action

An independent action is one in which each limb follows a different movement pathway (e.g. the sidestroke arm and leg actions).

Gliding (towards a streamlined body position)

Gliding skills must be consolidated before adding propulsion using the limbs. This can be introduced using flotation aids; then progressed to gliding independently.

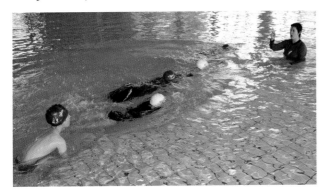

Gliding

PUSH AND GLIDE

Students push off from the bottom, side or steps of the pool. They should be encouraged to open their eyes, blow bubbles and let the legs float freely behind.

Teachers should get students to try gliding variations such as:

- with legs wide or together
- with legs curled
- without a flotation aid
- underwater.

Teachers should encourage students to experiment with body orientation and body steering skills by rotating during push and glide activities, for example:

- push and glide — rotate to the left side
- push and glide — rotate to the right side
- push and glide — rotate to either side and back to prone
- push and glide — perform a full 360 degree rotation.

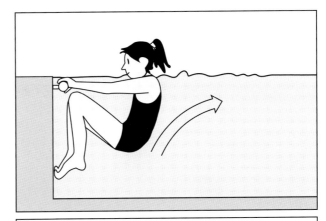

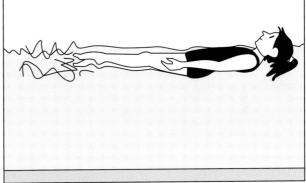

Push and glide on the back

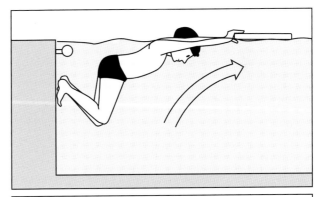

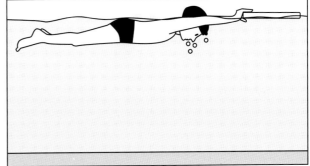

Push and glide on the front

PUSH AND GLIDE WITH KICK

Setting the task of using the legs and feet for propulsion, students move through the water, head first:

- on the water surface
- underwater (for a very short distance).

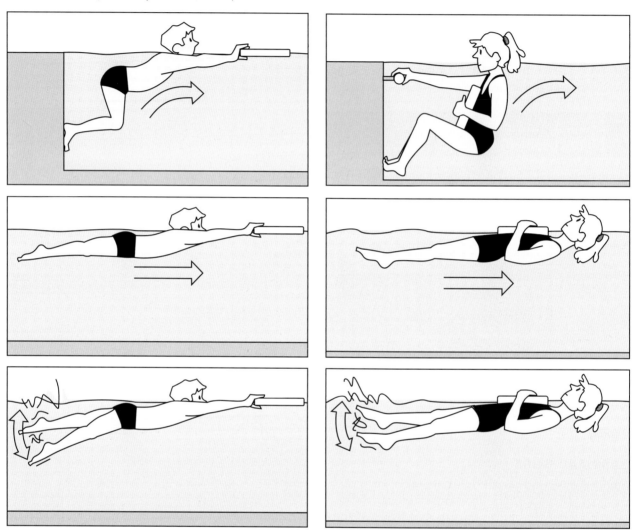

Push, glide, kick on front

Push, glide, kick on back

THE TORPEDO

The torpedo is a combination of a glide with an alternate (flutter) kick. Teachers should encourage students to use a relaxed leg action originating from the hips, with the legs long and loose (like kicking off your socks without the use of your hands). Students should try the torpedo on:

- the back
- the side.

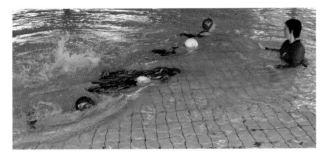

Torpedo

PUSH AND GLIDE WITH ARMS

Using the arms only, students should explore different ways to move through the water, head first, feet first and sideways:

- on the water surface
- underwater (for a very short distance).

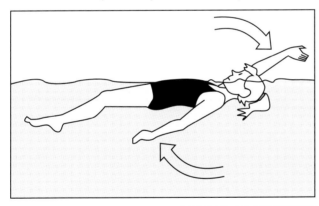

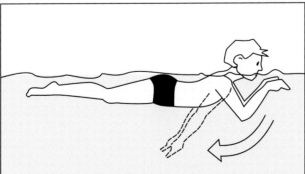

Propelling activities using the hands and arms

Propulsion/mobility experiences

The following activities can be done with or without a flotation aid.

- Push off from the wall, steps or bottom of the pool, and move the legs.
- Perform a different alternate, independent or paired leg action each time.
- Try the above activities on the back and side.
- Stop and compare the action, for example:
  - 'What action made the most splash?'
  - 'What action was the easiest?'
  - 'What action pushed you the longest distance?'

Beginners:

- use an alternate arm action to move head first through the water with both above-water and underwater arm recoveries
- use a paired arm action to move head first through the water with both above-water and underwater arm recoveries
- keep the arms near the side and find various ways of using the arms and hands to move head first and feet first — this activity can be tried with the arms held out beyond the head or underneath the body.

Students can also try the above activities on their back and their side.

> **TEACHING TIP**
> Encourage students to invent their own ways of moving through the water using alternate, independent and paired leg and arm actions with both above-water and underwater recoveries.

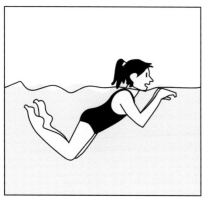
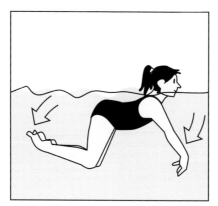
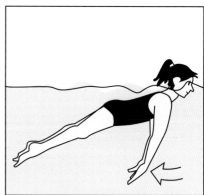
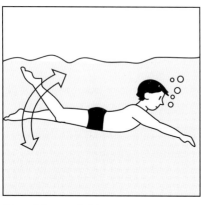
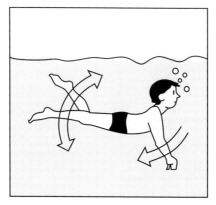
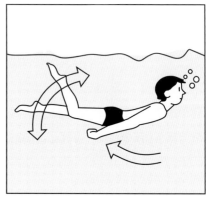

Propulsion activities

PROPULSION FORWARDS, BACKWARDS AND SIDEWAYS

Leg and arm actions are now combined to explore different ways of moving forwards, backwards or sideways on the surface and underwater.

Try the following propulsion/mobility actions:

- use combinations of paired arm and leg actions, with various recoveries and in various body positions
- use combinations of alternate arm and leg actions with various recoveries and in various body positions
- use different leg and arm actions, move head first, feet first or sideways in a circle
- use alternate arm and leg actions to move head first — do four alternate arm actions on the front (face down) then roll onto the back and repeat (breathing while on the back, blowing bubbles while on the front)
- try the above using paired arm and leg actions
- propel through submerged hoops or through a partner's legs
- submerge and use the legs and arms to return to the surface feet first, head first or sideways
- return to the surface vertically or sideways, head first and assume different body shapes, from an underwater position.

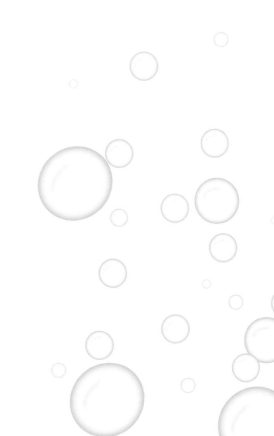

BREATHING ACTIVITIES

During the water familiarisation stage, breathing activities were introduced. Now that students are more confident in their mobility skills, more advanced breathing activities can be introduced. Students can:

- walk and inhale, then submerge and exhale (every three steps)
- while standing, turn the head to one side (one ear in the water) and inhale, then roll the face into the water and exhale
- walk with hands behind the back and the face in the water, turn so one ear is in the water, inhale, then, on rolling the face back into the water, exhale
- try the above activities while doing different arm actions (e.g. push, glide, kick with arms while breathing)

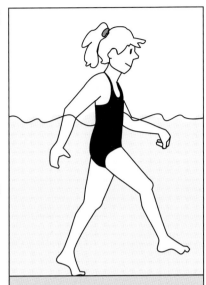 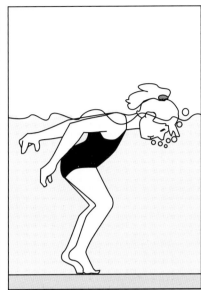

Breathing practice and walking

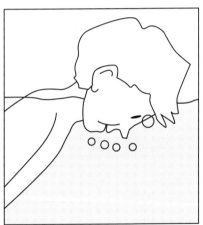 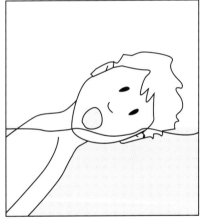

Breathing practice while rotating the head to the side

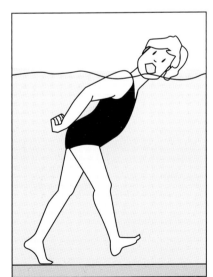 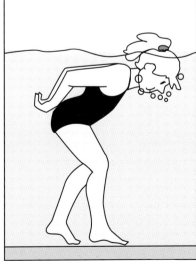

Breathing practice while walking and turning the head to the side

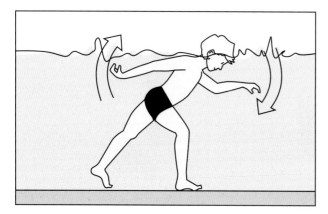

Breathing practice with different arm actions

- using a flotation aid for support, kick across the pool, completing the breathing actions on the right side, then the left side

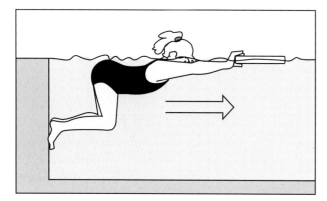

Breathing action with a flotation aid

- using different arm and leg actions, try breathing to the front (as in breaststroke).

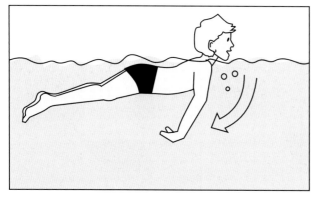

Breathing action with different limb movements

For students who are too busy concentrating on the arm action and breathing to remember to kick the legs, a flotation aid may be useful.

Distances should gradually be increased and a rhythmical breathing action encouraged.

Sculling

Sculling is the basic skill upon which all strokes and many other techniques are based. Sculling movements resemble the action of a ship's screw propeller and involve changing the pitch of the hands for the most effective propulsion through the water or for the maintenance of a stable body position.

When developing sound sculling technique it is important to remember that the back of the hand faces the direction of preferred travel.

Below are progressions which students can follow in developing the sculling technique.

ON THE EDGE OF THE POOL OR FLAT SURFACE

While standing in the water with the arms initially out of the water:

- angle palms out with little finger leading (outward sweep)
- angle palms in with thumbs leading (inward sweep).

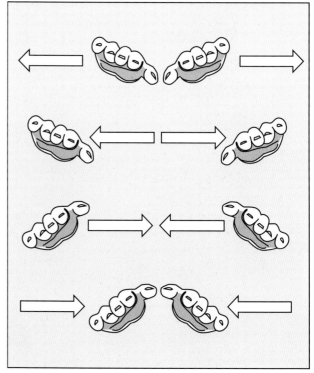

Sculling action

STANDING IN SHALLOW WATER

Standing in shallow water, beginners can:

- practise the outward and inward sweep of the sculling action just under the surface of the water
- keep the upper arms reasonably still and allow the hands and forearms to move outwards and inwards in relaxed, smooth but firm, continuous movements.

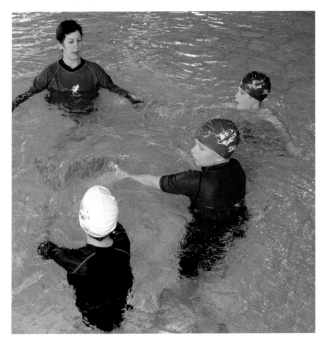

Standing in shallow water, sculling

SHOULDER-DEEP WATER

Standing in shoulder-deep water and sculling, beginners can bend both knees and lift the feet gently off the bottom of the pool. The lifting effect of the scull can be improved by increasing the speed of the action.

TEACHING TIP
Encourage students to apply equal pressure against the water for both the outward and inward sculling sweeps.

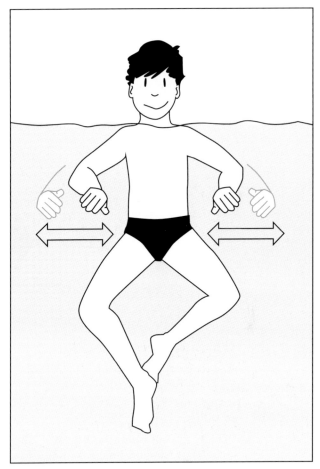

Standing in shoulder-deep water, sculling

SCULLING CHECKLIST
- ❑ Hands are relatively flat (not cupped).
- ❑ Hands are angled at 45 degrees.
- ❑ Horizontal outward and inward movements of the hands.
- ❑ Upper arms are relatively still.
- ❑ Action is relaxed, smooth, firm and continuous.

Students can practise sculling while in a tucked position, using the hands alternately to rotate the body.

TYPES OF SCULLING

Stationary sculling (flat sculling)

Stationary sculling is used to maintain a stationary position and to gain lift. This is achieved by holding the fingertips at the same level as the wrist.

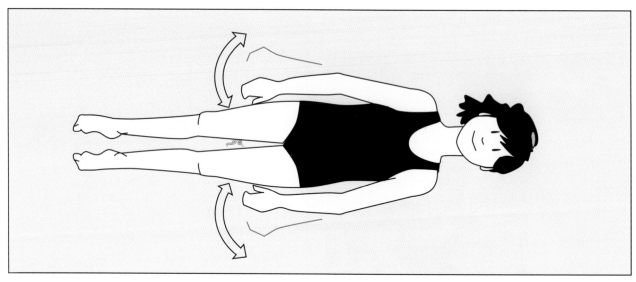

Stationary sculling

Head-first sculling

The arms are held by the sides and a back-float position is adopted. The hand position is with the fingertips tilted up towards the surface of the water.

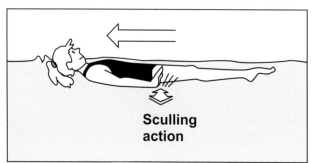

Head-first sculling

Feet-first sculling

For feet-first sculling the above position is adopted and the fingertips are tilted down towards the bottom of the pool.

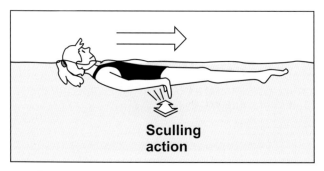

Feet-first sculling

SAFETY SKILLS

It is important that basic safety skills and rescue knowledge be introduced to students as early as possible. The 'bare basics' are outlined here, but are covered in detail in further chapters.

Basic safety skills include:

- knowledge and understanding of class and pool rules
- knowledge and understanding of basic personal safety rules including:
  - never swimming alone
  - letting someone know before you get into water
  - checking it is safe before getting into water.

Basic rescue skills

Students should be introduced to knowledge and skills associated with rescues including the following.

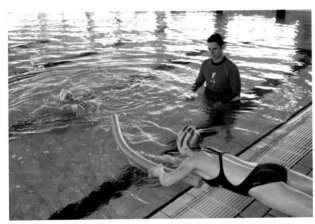

Reach out to partner with a rigid aid (pole, hoop) or non-rigid aid (towel, clothing) to pull them in

Partner grasps the aid with one or two hands and is pulled into the edge

Keep the body as low as possible when pulling in a person in difficulty

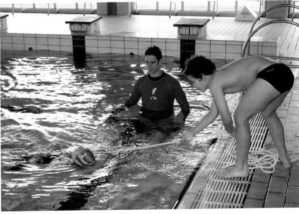

Throw a flotation aid to partner (or into floating hoop), such as:

- *an unweighted rope*
- *a weighted rope — use rope dipped into water to give it 'weight'*
- *a kickboard*
- *a ball*
- *a plastic bottle*

Ensure feet are apart and firmly placed when throwing

Person in difficulty should experience being rescued on their back, side and front

Water safety activities

Water safety activities at this stage should reinforce students' skills in combining the use of buoyancy aids with the alternative methods of propulsion to assist in performing a self-rescue. To practise water safety, students:

- using the arms, legs, or arms and legs, move to a floating buoyant rescue aid
- submerge and surface next to a buoyancy aid
- pretend that they have been injured and, using an aid thrown to them, propel themselves to the edge of the pool (e.g. using only one arm)
- pretend that they are in deep water, float on the back with an aid and then kick to the edge
- practise putting on a personal flotation device (PFD) in the water
- while wearing a PFD, try various arm and leg swimming actions.

WATER SAFETY ACTIVITIES USING FLOTATION AIDS

'Reach-to-rescue' skills can be introduced in games and fun activities and can be expanded to include the use of flotation aids and students' buoyancy skills. For example, students:

- use a flotation aid to float in various positions, then on a signal, kick to the edge and climb out
- enter the water while holding a flotation aid, float and then return to the edge
- throw a flotation aid to a partner, instruct them to float on the back or front then kick to the edge
- enter the water wearing a PFD
- float, roll over and try different types of propulsion while wearing the PFD.

INTRODUCTION TO DEEPER WATER

Eventually, the time comes when teachers must decide whether their students are ready to be introduced to deeper water. Water is considered deeper when students cannot stand on the bottom with the mouth clear of the surface.

Some students are enthusiastic, others may be apprehensive about the thought of deeper water even though they feel confident in the water.

Some teachers believe in introducing deep-water activities very early in the program. Others want the students to be able to float. Others again require that students be able to propel themselves for a certain distance before they allow them to experience deeper water. The time is right when teachers decide the moment has come for their particular class! Teachers should know the individual characteristics of the students and what their students can cope with. However, safety, encouragement and patience are the key words for deeper-water experience activities.

It is important that students are aware that when they submerge vertically into water, care should be taken to avoid water being forced up the nostrils. The blowing of 'nose bubbles' should be encouraged at all times.

DEEPER-WATER ACTIVITIES INCLUDE:

- walk hand over hand along the wall (crab crawling) from the shallow end to the deep end
- submerge slowly, while holding the edge with hands, until the arms are fully extended
- bob up and down while holding the edge and blowing nose bubbles
- face the edge and relax, letting legs hang, then take a breath and put the face into the water (to look at the feet)
- submerge while holding onto the edge with one hand only
- facing the edge with chins in the water, take a breath then let go of the edge and let their bodies sink (vertical float)
- try the vertical float with arms above the head
- submerge (while close to the wall), touch the bottom and push off to resurface. This activity should be started in water that is not too deep.
- play 'Fireman's Pole' — climbing down the pole feet first until the feet touch the bottom and, as confidence grows, climbing down and picking up an object
- jump in, surface and grasp a noodle held by the teacher (it may be held one to two metres away if the teacher knows that students will move towards it)
- jump in and move unassisted to the side, with the noodle held nearby should it be needed
- float using a flotation aid (e.g. a PFD).

Treading water

Treading water can be very tiring for students, and teachers should take all safety precautions into consideration when teaching this skill.

Students can practise treading water:

- holding onto the edge with one hand
- using a flotation device
- holding a flotation aid
- using a PFD
- when close to the edge of the pool
- with horizontal arm sculling
- using different leg actions (e.g. flutter kick, breaststroke kick, scissor kick, egg beater kick).

GAMES

Games make learning an enjoyable experience and help students learn water skills through play. Appendix 6 includes some games and activities that teachers may use. There are many other land-based games and activities that can be adapted for the water. When conducting games in water, teachers should consider the age and ability of each group member, the number of participants, water space and conditions, and the availability of equipment.

TEACHING TIP
Games shouldn't be used simply to fill in time before a lesson ends. Use a game to reinforce a particular skill you have just taught the students — they will be learning without actually realising it!

SAMPLE LESSON PLAN ACTIVITIES

The first contact that students have with the water should be an active, enjoyable, fun experience.

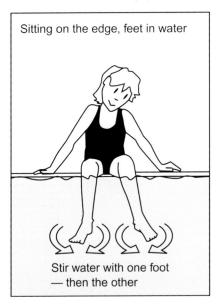

Sitting on the edge, feet in water

Stir water with one foot — then the other

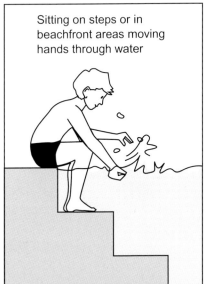

Sitting on steps or in beachfront areas moving hands through water

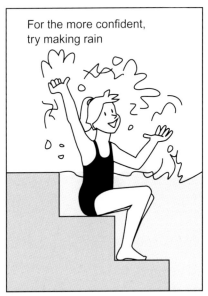

For the more confident, try making rain

First experience — let's get wet

Entries and exits

The how, why and when of entries into the water should be discussed with students:

- how to perform the entries with safety (refer to Chapter 5, 'Aquatic safety, survival and rescue skills', for detailed information on entries)
- why certain entries are used (e.g. 'step in' is used when the water is clear, the depth known and the bottom clear of obstacles)

- when to use certain entries (e.g. dive into deep water)
- jump into the water wearing a PFD
- slide in, pretend there is an obstacle and climb back out
- do a sitting dive, float or tread water, then swim unassisted to the edge and climb out
- catch a flotation aid thrown by the teacher and use it to kick back to the edge and climb out.

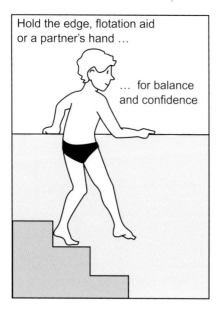

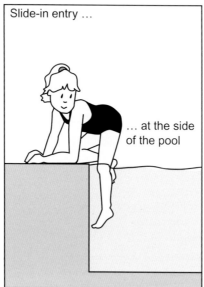

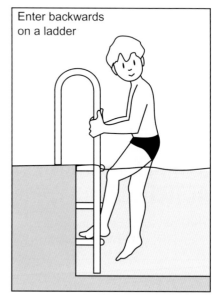

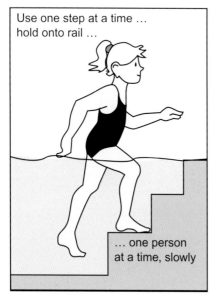

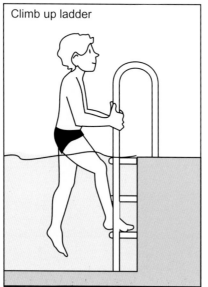

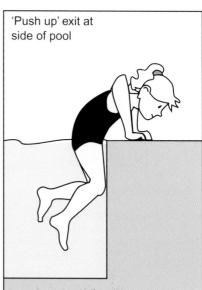

Entering and exiting the water

Safety for the student and others is of utmost importance.

Standing and moving through the water

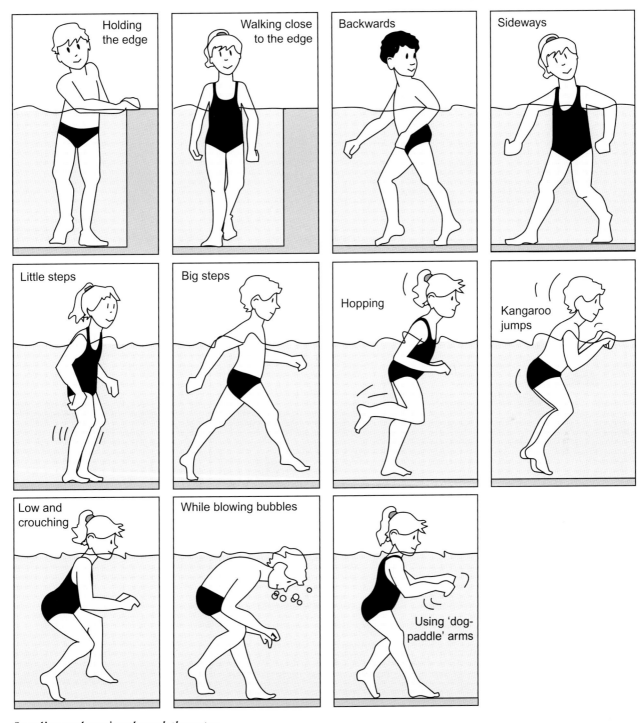

Standing and moving through the water

Students should first become familiar with moving vertically through the water, before they progress to moving horizontally.

Getting the face wet

Getting the face wet is an important progression before submerging.

Washing face, hair

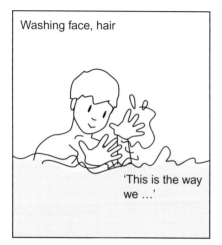

'This is the way we ...'

Making rain

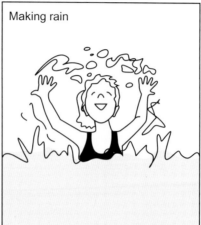

Catch and throw ball with partner

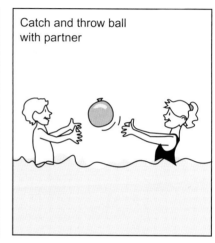

Under the shower

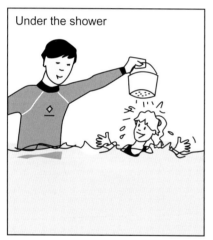

Splashball

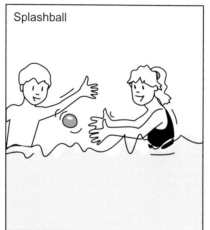

Scoop and pour over partner's head

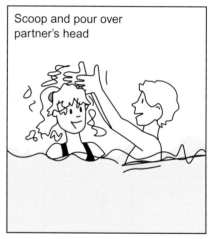

Getting the face wet

TEACHING TIP
Get students to place their forehead in the water first. Don't go straight down like a lift descending as water will go right up the nose — ouch!

Submerging

'Ring a ring o' roses' —
a great start to a lesson

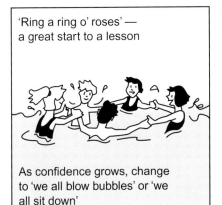

As confidence grows, change
to 'we all blow bubbles' or 'we
all sit down'

Ducking under hoops

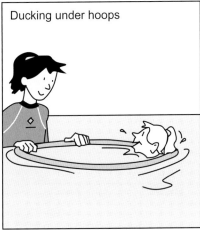

Bob under to touch

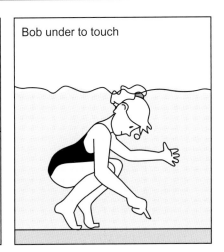

Pick up objects

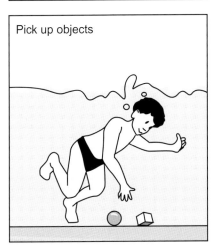

Climb down a
broomstick to touch
the bottom, or sit on
bottom of pool

Monkey stick

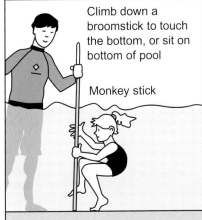

Submerge while
holding partner
or side of pool

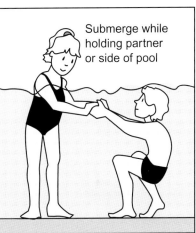

Submerging

Fun activities and games are essential in learning.

Opening eyes underwater

Look at hands and feet underwater	Count a partner's fingers	Watch a partner's bubbles, or make faces
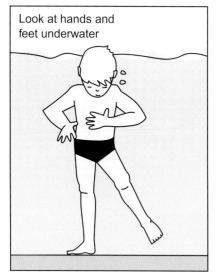	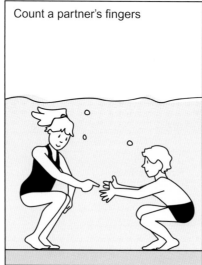	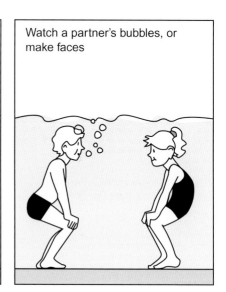

Pick up a certain colour ring or object	Waterproof flashcards with different actions
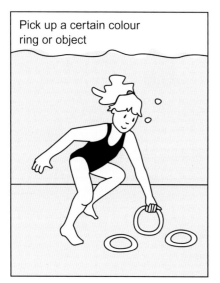	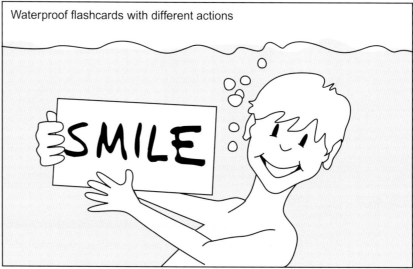

Opening eyes underwater — an essential progression to become familiar with the water

Recovery to a standing position — from front float

The aim is to be able to return to a safe, stable standing position.

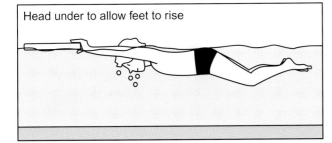

Head under to allow feet to rise

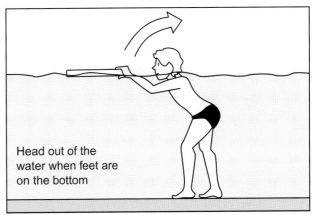

Head out of the water when feet are on the bottom

Recovery to a standing position — from front float

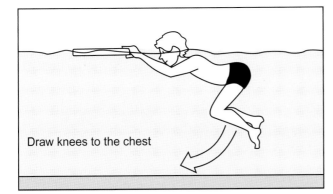

Draw knees to the chest

Recovery to a standing position — from back float

The aim is to be able to return to a safe, stable standing position.

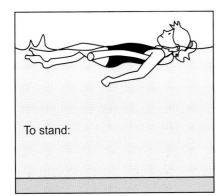

To stand:

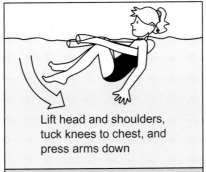

Lift head and shoulders, tuck knees to chest, and press arms down

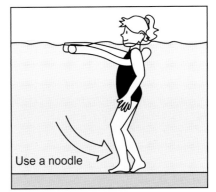

Use a noodle

Recovery to a standing position — from back float

Breathing activities

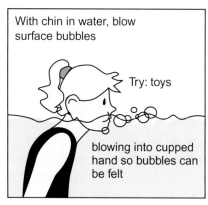

With chin in water, blow surface bubbles

Try: toys

blowing into cupped hand so bubbles can be felt

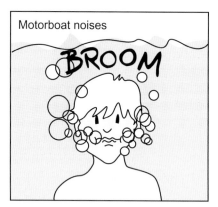

Motorboat noises

BROOM

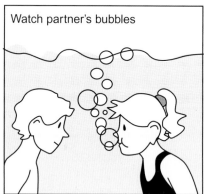

Watch partner's bubbles

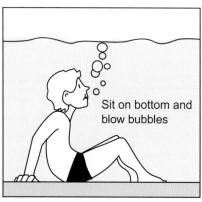

Sit on bottom and blow bubbles

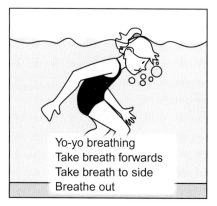

Yo-yo breathing
Take breath forwards
Take breath to side
Breathe out

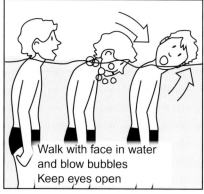

Walk with face in water and blow bubbles
Keep eyes open

Breathing activities

Breathing activities should be constantly reinforced with all practices.

REVIEW QUESTIONS

1   What should the aim of your swimming and water safety program be?
2   Discuss the students' needs and explain their importance when introducing a student to the aquatic environment.
3   What are the factors relating to the 'human body in water' that are important for a teacher to understand before familiarising students with water?
4   Discuss how skills in floating on the front and the back can be introduced to students.
5   List as many different activities you can think of that will assist with developing skills in:
    * water familiarisation
    * buoyancy and mobility
    * safety.

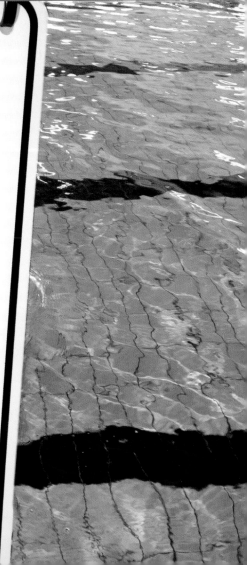

SHALLOW
WATER
NO
DIVING

INTRODUCTION

Every year, about 25 young Australians become quadriplegics as a result of diving into shallow water. Typically, the injured person is an athletic male aged between 15 and 29 years. His diving skills are usually self-taught and he is unaware of the potential dangers associated with diving into shallow water and the skills required to perform low-risk dive entries. Often alcohol consumption has been associated with the injury.

Swimming and water safety teachers and coaches play a vital role in the prevention of spinal cord injury caused in diving accidents. They must alert students to the potential dangers inherent in diving and assist students in acquiring the skills to improve diving safety. It must be emphasised that diving is only one way to enter the water, and perhaps the least preferred from a safety perspective. A dive entry should be used *only* when the condition of the water is known to be deep and free of obstacles. Slide-in and wade-in entries are the only safe ways to enter water when depth is unknown or obstacles could be present.

In water familiarisation programs, students are exposed to many new water experiences. Activities involving submerging, lifting feet from the bottom and entering the water via slide-in occur in the early learning phase. Lead-up skills for low-risk dives should also be incorporated very early in swimming and water safety programs. Gliding and steering skills, which are vital to the performance of low-risk dives, should form part of basic body orientation and water awareness activities. The progressions included later in this chapter illustrate the skills to be incorporated.

SKILLS FOR SAFER DIVING — LOCK HANDS, LOCK HEAD, STEER UP

In a study comparing 'low-risk' and 'high-risk' dives, several factors were found to contribute to safer dive entries. Safer dives are shallower, with hands held together and arms extended beyond the head, thus offering protection against impact. Locking hands together is important to prevent the arms being forced apart or deliberately pulled apart upon impact with the water. Arms must remain extended beyond the head until the student is well into the upward phase of the underwater pathway. Observation of dives performed by people with a low level of diving skill shows that often these people increase the potential risk of injury when they pull both arms backward in a breaststroke-like action during the downward phase of their underwater pathway. To prevent this occurrence, the hands must remain locked together. This can be achieved by placing one hand on top of the other, with the thumb and little finger of the top hand wrapped around the sides of the bottom hand. The thumb of the bottom hand should squeeze against the little finger of the top hand. The teaching cue '*lock hands*' should be used.

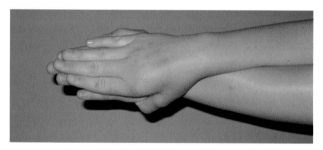

Lock hands

Diving safety is further enhanced when the head is squeezed between the outstretched arms, with the pressure of the arms ensuring that the head is locked in this position. In this '*lock head*' position, the head is fixed in place between the arms to prevent sideways movement of the neck. By locking the head in this way, the vertebrae of the neck are aligned and the spinal cord is well protected. The spinal cord is more vulnerable if impact occurs when the vertebrae of the neck are twisted or turned in any way. Some spinal cord injuries occur without contact with the bottom, and in fact result from impact with the water when the vertebrae of the neck are not carefully aligned. The cue *lock head* acts to reinforce and remind students of the correct alignment of the spine to minimise the risk of injury.

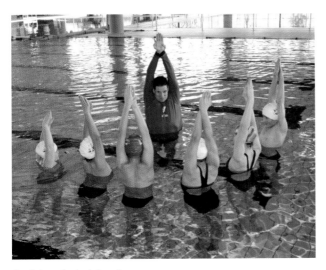

Lock hands, lock head

The underwater pathway of a dive is significantly influenced by the implementation of steering-up skills. '*Steering up*' refers to using body and limb angles so that the student's pathway is towards the surface. To aid steering up towards the surface, students should bend back the hands at the wrists, raise the upper trunk, arch the back, lift the head and raise the arms. These actions should be employed very early in the underwater pathway. When steering-up skills are used, the maximum depth reached is shallower and occurs earlier in the underwater pathway. Students should receive constant reminders to '*steer up*'.

TEACHING TIP
Remember to constantly remind your students to 'steer up'.

Flight distance and entry angle also affect the depth of a dive. Students, even while learning, should aim for good horizontal velocity and a long flight. By aiming to enter the water at a greater distance from the edge, flight distance is increased and entry angle is decreased. Many students who lack confidence do not push outwards (horizontally) hard enough and enter the water very close to the edge, using a steep entry angle. This results in a deeper, higher-risk dive. With increased flight, both entry angle and dive depth are decreased, resulting in a lower risk dive. One way of increasing flight distance is to ask students to jump into the water, as far out from the edge as possible. Then, when performing a dive entry, they should aim to enter the water at the same distance as their entry point when jumping.

Another method of increasing flight distance is to place a small buoyant object, such as a piece of foam about 10 cm square, on the surface of the water at the point where the student's hands should enter. The student then aims to touch the foam as they enter the water.

A spinal injury can occur when a student slips on the pool decking, and subsequently does not have sufficient horizontal velocity and consequently performs a deep dive with a very steep entry angle. To prevent this occurrence, teachers should insist that students curl their toes over the lip of the pool when performing a dive entry. This enables the students to prevent the steep dive that follows slipping as, even if the decking is wet, it is still possible to push backwards against the edge of the pool, hence providing horizontal force for flight. Toes should curl over the pool edge for every dive entry.

TEACHING TIP
Get your students to curl their toes over the edge every time they perform a dive entry — this will help to prevent slipping.

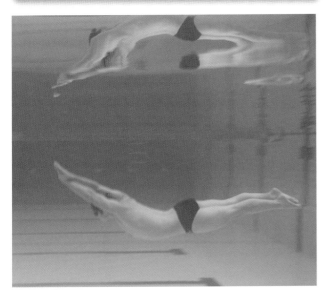

Lock hands, lock head, steer up

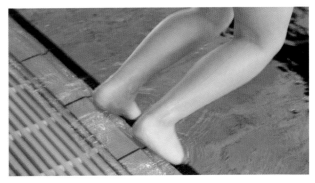

Toes curled over edge

The cues *lock hands*, *lock head* and *steer up* should be continually reinforced throughout diving instruction whether with beginning students or when refining the diving skills of more experienced students. Implementation of these actions will result in safer dive entries.

When teaching diving skills, swimming and water safety teachers have the responsibility to convey the importance of checking that the water is deep and free of obstacles prior to performing any head-first entry. It is relevant to note that the velocity achieved during virtually all dive entries is sufficient to dislocate or crush the vertebrae of the neck. Hence, the utmost caution must be exercised for every head-first entry in an effort to prevent serious and permanent injury, which can result from just one poorly executed dive.

> **TEACHING TIP**
> Exercise the utmost caution when your students are diving.

TEACHING PROGRESSIONS FOR SAFER DIVING SKILLS

The first progression for safer diving skills should start very early in water confidence classes. Gliding and steering-up skills can be introduced as soon as students are confident to submerge their face. They can be safely conducted in shallow water because they are performed following a push from the wall, rather than a head-first entry from the edge. Teachers should establish the *lock hands, lock head* position from the initial introduction of gliding skills. Throughout all gliding and steering-up skills outlined in these progressions, the student *does not* kick with the legs or pull with the arms.

1. Push to glide

Students should adopt the *lock hands, lock head* position, completely submerge and then push off from the wall. In the first instance, the arms and body should be held straight, and the glide will be straight ahead, in a streamlined position. There should be no kicking of legs or pulling of arms. During this 'push to glide', students should look down, towards the bottom of the pool, keeping their chin tucked toward the chest.

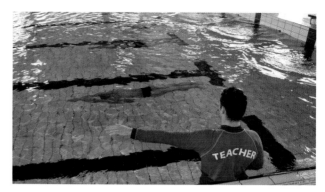

Push to glide

2. Push to glide, steering up

Following the successful achievement of the 'push to glide' skill, steering up should be introduced. This progression commences in the same way as 'push to glide' (lock hands, lock head, then submerge and push off the wall) but upon departure from the wall, the student steers up towards the surface. To achieve this, students change the angle of the wrists and upper body. Pointing fingertips upwards, arching the back and lifting the head slightly enables them to steer up towards the surface. Hands and head should remain locked until the hands break through the surface. This prevents students performing the unsafe breaststroke-like arm action typical of some high-risk dives.

To enhance water awareness, students should also experience changing their body position to travel downwards. While this is a most undesirable action in diving, its inclusion in the gliding activities from the wall provides students with a greater understanding of how body position affects underwater pathway. Hence, a small amount of time should be spent on steering the body down towards the bottom of the pool. To experience this, with hands locked and head locked, students should push off the wall, then point the fingertips downwards and curve the head and neck down. This will act to steer the student down, towards the bottom of the pool.

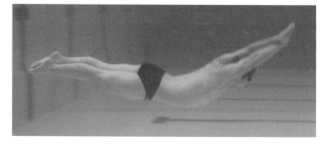

Push to glide, steering up

3. Glide through hoop tunnel

To further improve steering-up skills and to add extra fun, the third progression involves gliding through a hoop tunnel. In this instance, students push off the wall with hands locked and head locked, then glide in a streamlined position, steering the body through hoops placed at various levels in the water. The aim is to use steering-up skills to achieve the appropriate pathway. Students *do not* kick or pull, but follow the desired pathway by use of hand, arm and body position. Hoops should be placed so that the hoop closest to the wall touches the bottom, the second hoop is halfway between the bottom and the surface, and the top of the third hoop touches the surface. Students then steer up through the hoops, towards the surface. This progression requires other students to hold hoops in the appropriate position when it is not their turn to glide.

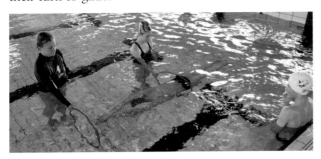

Push to glide through hoop tunnel

Following success with steering up through the hoops, the position of the third hoop should be changed, so that it is held horizontally on the surface of the water. Students push off the wall, steer up through the hoops to surface through the third hoop, with hands still locked together. Again, the cues *lock hands, lock head and steer up* must be emphasised. This progression is important to reinforce the necessity to surface with hands still locked together.

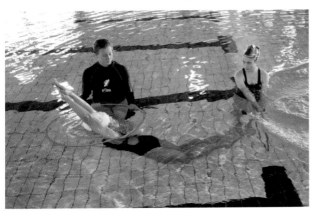

Push to glide, surface through hoop

4. Noodles and hoops

The first two hoops are replaced with noodles for this progression. Noodles are held horizontally on the water's surface. The student begins from standing alongside the first noodle, pushes off from the bottom of the pool and performs a dolphin-like action to spring over the first noodle, then steers under the second noodle, to surface through the horizontal hoop. The teacher should remind students to *lock hands, lock head and steer up*.

Once students are able to control their pathway through the water, they are ready to move to deep water and work through the more traditional diving progressions. As they have already developed skills which can be transferred to diving, it is likely that they will move through the traditional diving progressions more quickly than would be the case without the earlier progressions. Again, the cues *lock hands, lock head and steer up* must be emphasised.

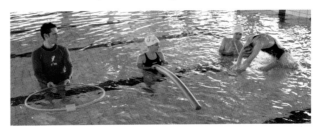

Noodles and hoop set up

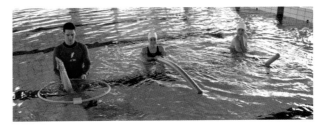

Noodles and hoop finish

5. Sit dive

The next progression — the sit dive — is a crucial step towards low-risk diving. Students sit on the pool edge, with their feet against the pool wall. With hands and head locked, they 'dive' into the water. Feet *must push back* against the pool wall. The action of pushing back against the wall with the feet prepares students for developing a long flight distance through the air when they move on to the next progression, the crouch dive. After entering the water, students should steer up. Teachers should spend a lot of time on this progression. With mastery of this skill, students will progress through the crouching and standing dives very quickly.

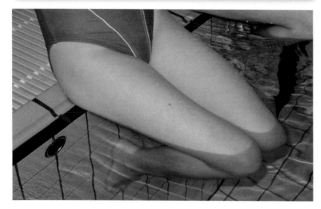

Sit dive — feet position

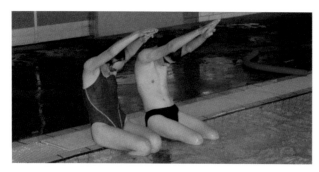

Sit dive — body start position

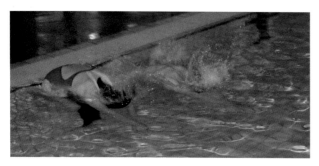

Sit dive — entry

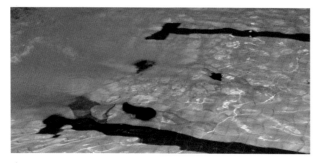

Sit dive — gliding

6. Crouch dive

Prior to commencing the crouch dive, use the feet-first jump described earlier (refer page 115). This will allow students to determine where they should aim for their hands to enter the water when they perform the crouch dive. For the crouch dive, students crouch on the pool edge, with one foot forward and one back. The toes of the front foot must curl over the edge, and hands and head must be locked. Weight is transferred from the back foot to the front foot and students 'tip' forward into the water, pushing against the pool edge with their toes. Upon entry, steering-up skills are implemented. As students gain confidence, feet can be placed together (toes of both feet curling over the pool edge) and stance can become more upright.

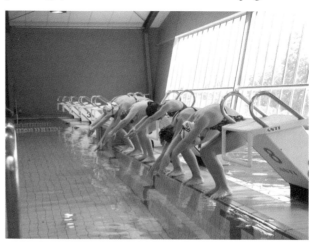

Crouch dive

7. Standing dive

Students stand with the toes of both feet curled over the pool edge. Initially the standing dive is performed just by tipping forward, with hands and head locked, and pushing with the toes against the pool edge. Hand-entry position should be at least as far as feet-entry position in the feet-first jump. Upon entry, steering up is applied.

For greater flight distance, ask students to dive over a soft foam mat. Flight distance will be increased as the student aims to clear the mat. Begin this activity with a short mat (or a longer mat placed sideways) and increase the length of the mat as the student increases flight distance with improved confidence. By using a soft mat, injury is avoided if a student does not completely clear the mat. Once students are confident and skilled in the standing dive, diving from starting blocks can also be included.

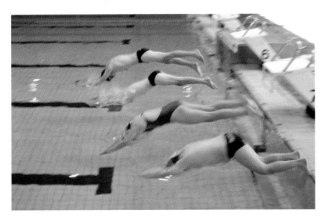

Standing dive

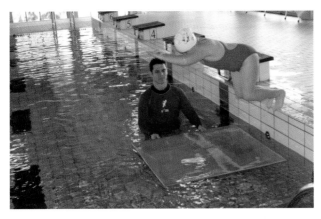

Diving over soft mat — beginner

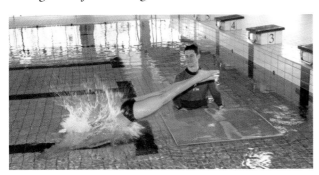

Diving over soft mat — advanced

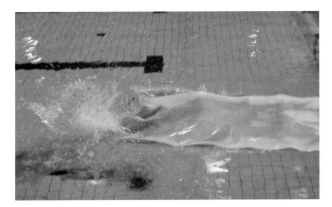

Diving over soft mat — safe foot contact

For progressions 6 and 7 (crouching and standing dives), water should be deep — preferably at least 2 m. However, water of this depth is not always available. It would be possible to perform these progressions in 1.5 m deep water, but it is recommended that signage be displayed to indicate that diving is occurring under instruction. In this circumstance, it is preferable to have the teacher in the water, standing alongside the point where the student's hands should enter the water. This will encourage the student to have a long flight distance, minimising the level of risk. Teachers must remain vigilant at all times, and must only allow students to move on to the crouch dive once mastery of the sit dive can be repeatedly demonstrated. The sit dive can be performed in water as shallow as 1.2 m, or even 1 m with extra care, as the underwater pathway for this progression is generally relatively shallow. No matter how deep the water is, constant reminders of *lock hands, lock head and steer up* must occur. It is of paramount importance that these cues are remembered by students.

TEACHING TIP
It is of paramount importance that the cues '*lock hands, lock head and steer up*' are remembered by students.

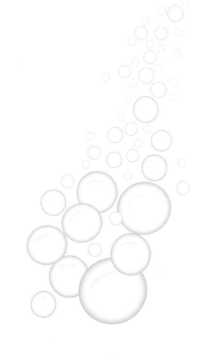

RULES FOR SAFE ENTRY

AUSTSWIM does not endorse the teaching of deep dives. It is not appropriate for teachers of swimming and water safety to teach students vertical entries for recreational diving. AUSTSWIM encourages the teaching of the shallow dive. Platform diving should always be taught and supervised by an appropriately qualified diving coach.

The previously mentioned water depths are to be used as a guide. For further information on guidelines relating to teaching of water entry and diving refer to the Royal Life Saving Society Australia *Guidelines for Safe Pool Operation*. The folder can be purchased off the internet at www.royallifesaving.com.au.

The following safety rules indicate the level of information required to assess a safe entry. It is recommended that teachers encourage alternative, safer entries.

- Slide in to check that the water depth is adequate before diving or jumping into unfamiliar bodies of water.
- Check for 'No diving' or 'No jumping' signs and obey them.
- Do not dive or slide head first into shallow water.
- Do not dive from structures not specifically designed for diving.
- Do not run and dive.
- Do not dive across the narrow part of a pool — it is safer to dive from the end.
- Backward dives or competition dives should only be performed by trained people from diving boards or diving platforms.
- Check regularly for changes in depth or water conditions if diving or jumping into naturally occurring bodies of water.

Students must be made aware of the dangers of diving into unknown pools, ponds, dams, rivers or creeks. Children enjoy jumping and diving in the water, so they must learn correct techniques when they are capable of performing them. It is vitally important to highlight the dangers of entries when teaching swimming and water safety to students.

REVIEW QUESTIONS

1. Who is typically most likely to be injured in a diving-related incident?
2. Explain the following terms, and why they are important in teaching safer diving:
   - lock hands
   - lock head
   - steer up.
3. How can hoops and noodles be used effectively to teach safe diving?
4. What are the benefits of the 'sit dive' progressions when teaching safer diving?
5. Explain the diving progressions from a crouch dive to a standing dive.
6. How deep should the water be when teaching diving?

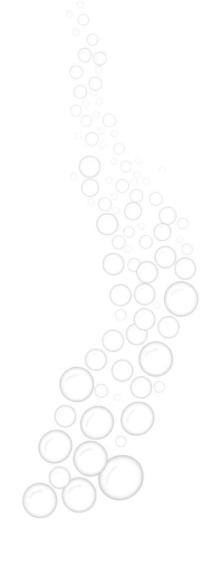

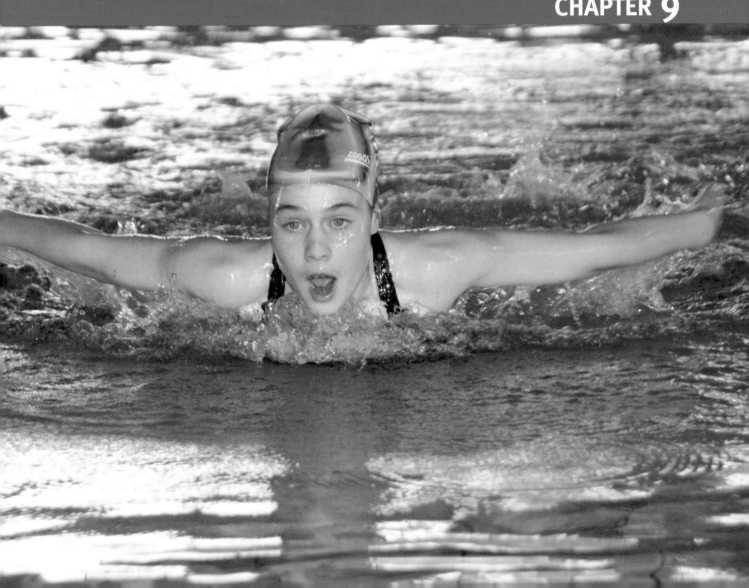

Towards efficient stroke development

CHAPTER 9

A BRIEF HISTORY

Australians have contributed greatly to the development of both the competitive and survival swimming strokes that are commonly used throughout the world today.

Freestyle

Freestyle, as it is known today, originated as the 'Australian Crawl' or 'Front Crawl' and has seen vast improvements in efficiency and immense increases in swimming speed with further refinements of the stroke in recent years.

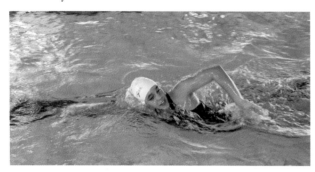

Freestyle

Backstroke

Backstroke developed from the basic back float, as people sought mobility while floating on their backs. This allowed them to be mobile without the need to learn complex breathing timing.

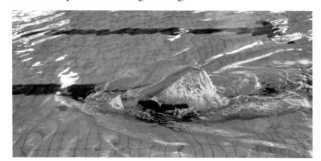

Backstroke

Breaststroke

It is believed that a form of breaststroke was the method first used to move the body in water. In many countries it is still taught today as the basis for all swimming.

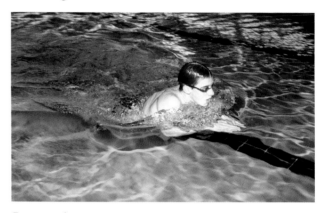

Breaststroke

Butterfly

Butterfly was derived through competition, as breaststrokers were looking to improve the speed of the stroke — over-water recovery of the arms was introduced to improve speed. Officials established butterfly as a competitive stroke and tightened the rules on breaststroke to prevent any form of outward over-water recovery of the arms.

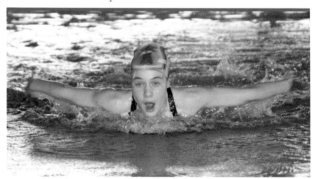

Butterfly

Sidestroke

Sidestroke is a useful technique for both personal survival and for the rescue of others. It is particularly suitable for rescues because the breathing and kicking actions are not hindered during towing. It also provides the benefit of not kicking the patient during a rescue.

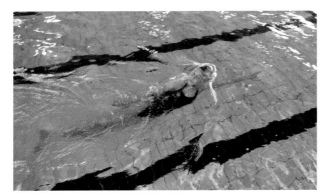

Sidestroke

Survival backstroke

Forms of survival backstroke are effective in both rescue and survival situations. The face is clear of the water, so breathing is uninterrupted and the inverted 'frog' or 'whip kick' is an efficient means of propulsion. A disadvantage of survival backstroke, however, is that the swimmer cannot see where they are going.

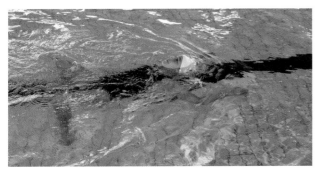

Survival backstroke

STROKE CHARACTERISTICS

Each stroke offers various advantages and is appropriate for various purposes.

FREESTYLE	BACKSTROKE
• competition	• competition
• rescue	• recreation
• recreation	• water polo
• water polo	
• prone board paddling	

BREASTSTROKE	BUTTERFLY
• competition	• competition
• rescue	• prone board paddling
• recreation	
• water polo	
• prone board paddling	

SIDESTROKE	SURVIVAL BACKSTROKE
• competition	• competition
• rescue	• rescue
• recreation	• recreation
• survival	• survival
• water polo	

The benefits that swimming provide are vast. Being able to swim can:
- provide you with an essential life skill
- develop essential safety skills and knowledge
- develop coordination
- provide other sporting and exercise opportunities (i.e. water skiing, hydrotherapy)
- enhance fitness level and body toning
- provide career opportunities.

Each of the strokes may be introduced to students in any order, depending on individual preferences and the circumstances of the aquatic environment. The objective of any instruction in any of the swimming strokes is to improve the mobility of students and increase their awareness of water safety. The development of appropriate and efficient skills is important to all students. Many of these basic skills are useful when learning all strokes.

The sequencing of skills is important — correct sequencing results in a more effective and efficient learning process. This also ensures that the skill is effectively reinforced and is efficiently reproduced in practice. The development of these skills must be based on an individual's own learning response and should be programmed to suit each individual student.

SWIMMING BASICS

Key skills

Mobility is the goal for students. To achieve a high level of mobility in the aquatic environment, students must develop the basic skills of water confidence, streamlining, recovery and various forms of propulsion.

These skills need to be taught in an easy-to-remember sequence that can be adopted as a basis for all swimming strokes. The sequence, once learnt, can then be the foundation for all future stroke development and can be reinforced as the strokes are further developed and refined. These basic mobility skills are of immense value to students at all levels of stroke development and continue through to competitive swimming and lifesaving.

The sequence that can be taught and retained at a young age is simple: submerge the face, push and glide, kick, arm stroke action and recovery. Breathing skills can be introduced as the skill is practised and further developed at a later stage.

> **SWIMMING SKILL SEQUENCE**
> Submerge the face, push and glide, kick, arm stroke action and recovery.

These skills must be taught and reinforced to create mobile students who can then develop other skills which may be further modified, adapted and refined as required.

These basic key learner skills (known as the basic learner sequence) are the basis for successful skill development and must be taught in an effective manner to result in a sound base of skill learning by students.

During the initial stroke development phase, students should experiment with three types of body positions:
1 face down — prone
2 face up — on back, supine
3 prone and turning face on side (breathing foundation skill).

Face immersion

While this skill is often one of the most difficult for students to acquire, time spent on teaching this skill is extremely valuable at all future learning stages. This skill must be practised in a variety of different water depths, temperatures and conditions (if available), to ensure that students are confident and that they have learnt the skill effectively. This needs to be practised with the head in all positions — as detailed below.

FACE-DOWN GLIDING POSITION

The means of developing a streamlined body position commences with students standing with feet slightly apart and knees bent to allow the shoulders to be under the water. The chin rests on the surface of the water and the arms extend forward, in a streamlined position.

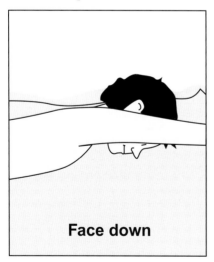

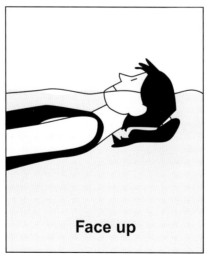

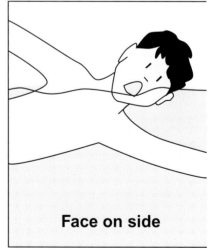

| Face down | Face up | Face on side |

Differences in body position

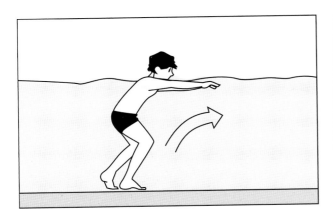

Face-down gliding position

Glide

Students take in a 'normal' volume of air and place the head into the water until approximately one-third of the skull area is in the water and the face is looking down and slightly forward. They push gently from the bottom into a streamlined position, indicated by the buttocks and the heels at the surface of the water. If the heels are not at the surface, the head should be positioned a little deeper into the water. Students can also practise the glide by placing one foot against the wall of the pool and pushing off.

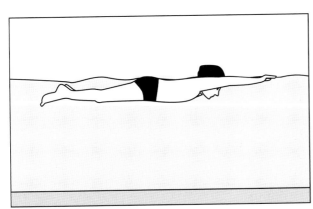

Streamlined position

Recovery

Following the glide, students should press the hands towards the bottom of the water while drawing the knees to the chest into a tuck position. The head should exit the water following the completion of the tucking action.

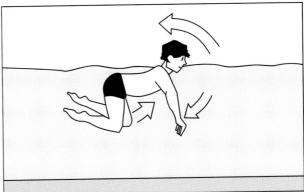

Recovery from a glide

FACE-UP GLIDING POSITION — WITH A BOARD

This skill is taught once students are confident in performing the face-down body position and glide.

Gliding position

Students stand with feet together and bend the knees to lower the shoulders into the water with the back of the head on the surface of the water.

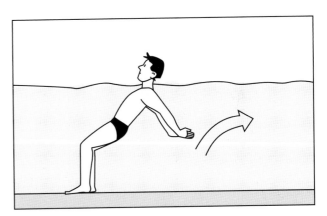

Starting position for a back glide

Glide

The glide is commenced by pushing off gently, with the ears just under the surface and the eyes looking upwards. The feet gently rise to the surface as the glide continues.

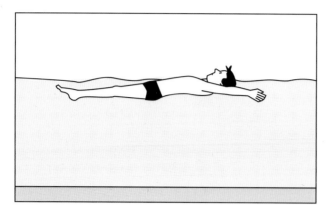

Back glide position

Recovery

Following the glide, the knees are drawn towards the chest while the head is brought towards the knees. Usually a great deal of water rushes over the student's head at this point — so the teacher needs to be prepared for this.

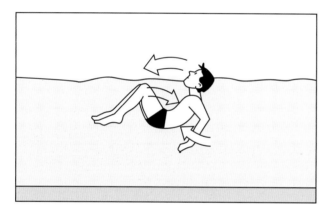

Recovery from a back glide

TEACHING TIP

If unfamiliar, the water rushing over a student's head can be distressing when recovering to a stand from a back glide or float — anticipate this and be prepared to help and reassure.

FACE ON THE SIDE — BREATHING POSITION

The body-on-side position is relatively easy to perform once students are competent at both the face-downward and face-upward body positions. Students should concentrate on keeping the lower ear in the water as they practise the glide.

Various glides with kick

Following the development of a streamlined body position, students may progress to the introduction of the kick. In time students should be encouraged to practise both competitive and survival kicking actions. The kick is a continuous action and requires a great deal of practice to master.

When initial practices for breaststroke and butterfly are being performed, the push from the bottom should commence with the feet together to encourage the development of the desired symmetrical action.

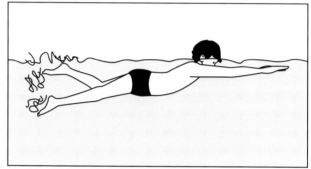

Gliding with a kick

THE SWIMMING STROKES

Information on all main swimming strokes follows. At the end of each specific stroke section you will find specific teaching progressions that relate to that stroke. Suggested steps are supported by notes made in point form in order to provide a simple quick reference for teachers.

There are many drills which have gained acceptance in developing particular aspects of the strokes.

The drills listed in the 'suggested steps' are tried, tested and known to be effective. However, there are many other drills and strategies which can be successfully employed.

In order to avoid confusing students when moving from one class to another, it is recommended that a common approach to the introduction of progressive drills and skills should be adopted by all teachers within any particular program.

FREESTYLE

Once the basic sequence has been developed and the skill of kick and recovery taught, then the skills of stroke and breathing can be introduced.

Body position

The body is in a prone position with the head raised slightly so the water is passing the forehead with the hips and legs just under the surface

Leg action

The common term for the freestyle kick is the 'flutter' kick, as the feet appear to flutter at the surface. The legs should be relaxed and the movement begins at the top of the legs. The leg flexes slightly at the knee prior to the down-beat and then straightens on the up-beat. Plantar-flexion (toe moves away from shin, like a ballet dancer pointing their toes) of the feet is important in the freestyle kick, but it should be the pressure of the water that plantar-flexes the foot, not the straining of the student. The action should be smooth and continuous.

Arm action

Before actually teaching the freestyle arm action it is important for teachers to have a sound understanding of the correct technique and its components.

The freestyle arm action is made up of a series of components. They are listed here and occur in an integrated sequence.

ENTRY

- The hand entry into the water must be smooth with a relatively high elbow and a raised wrist, the fingers and the hand entering the water first.
- Entry should be made approximately on the 'shoulder line'.
- The index finger and thumb should lead as the hand enters the water. After the entry, the hand pushes forward and slightly downwards. As the elbow reaches the extended position, the other hand is completing its propulsive pushing action under the hips.

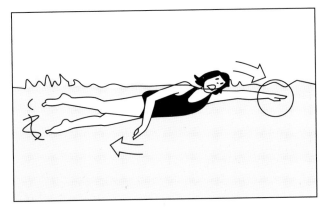

Hand entry position

CATCH

- The catch is made following the entry of the hand.
- The catch is the initial part of the pull and is performed with the wrist slightly flexed.
- The little finger leads the hand in a slight outward sweep which applies force against the water and assists in propelling the body forward.

The entry and catch components of all strokes are considered by many to be the most important aspects of the stroke.

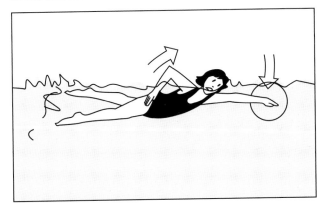

Hand catch position

PULL

- At the completion of the catch, the elbow has begun to flex and the hand begins a downward and outward pathway — **downsweep**.
- The elbow continues to flex throughout the downsweep.
- As the hand approaches its deepest point, the downsweep is rounded off into an **insweep**, with the elbow flexed to right angles and the arm continuing in this position under the shoulders.

PUSH

- The push phase commences at the end of the insweep. This is approximately under the student's chest. Remember that the body rolls during this action.
- During the propulsive push phase, the hand moves backwards, outwards and upwards.
- Pressure created by this action propels the body forward.
- Once the hip has moved over the hand, pressure against the palm of the hand is released slightly and the elbow begins to flex to allow the hand to leave the water smoothly.

The push phase is considered by many to be the most propulsive part of the arm stroke.

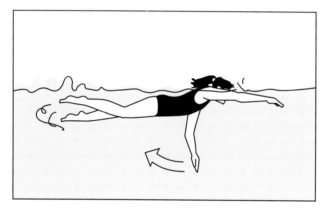

Hand push position

RECOVERY

- The desired arm recovery is with a high elbow action initiated by a roll of the shoulder with the hand passing close to the side of the body. The recovery commences at the end of the upward push movement of the hand.
- The upper arm/shoulder initiates the recovery and the elbow is raised. When the hand is clear of the water the arm rotates forward.
- The hand travels upwards, slightly outwards and forward during the first half of the recovery with the palm facing either inwards or backwards.
- The arm then extends forward and downwards as the index finger and thumb slide gracefully into the water for the next catch.

TEACHING TIP
The whole-skill teaching method is the best to use when introducing arm strokes. Only when students have difficulty with skills or require further development should the skill be taught in individual parts.

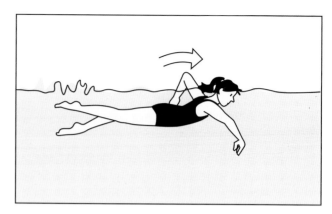

Hand recovery position

Breathing

TIMING
Before the timing of the arm action to the breathing pattern can be taught, it is essential that students develop an efficient breathing movement pattern. The following drills may assist.

The student while standing:
- holds a kickboard with both hands, thumb underneath and the fingers on top and elbows extended
- bends the knees to allow the shoulders to be under the water, turns the head to the side and places the face flat onto the water
- breathes in naturally and gently rotates the head until the eyes are facing the bottom of the pool. Without a pause they gently rotate the head out again.

During the inward and outward rotation, exhalation should occur through the mouth and nose.

Using a kickboard, students do a catch-up stroke. Each time the hand reaches the board to replace the other hand, students lean on that reaching hand and immediately turn the head to the opposite side to take a breath (inhale). They then complete another stroke cycle before repeating the sequence.

TEACHING TIP
Avoid over-practice of this drill as it may affect the student's natural stroke.

This activity promotes a relaxed and early breathing sequence that can be adapted to suit each individual. When introducing breathing timing, many teachers ask students to count the strokes and then turn the head to breathe. A common past method of teaching bilateral breathing had students count 1–2–3 and then turn the head to breathe, then count 1–2–3 and continue in that sequence. However, this method develops late breathing (which often results in student's lifting their head from the water to breathe) and should be avoided.

A more efficient method is to have students count 1–2 as each hand enters the water and, as the hand enters for the third stroke, they turn the head for the breath (i.e. 1–2–breathe, 1–2–breathe on the opposite side). This provides the support of the hand that has just entered the water for the learner to lean on. This also creates a cued sequence where there is a response for each action.

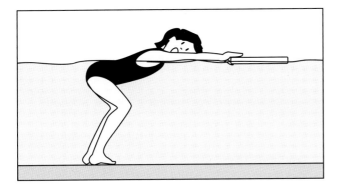

Breathing to the side in a stationary position

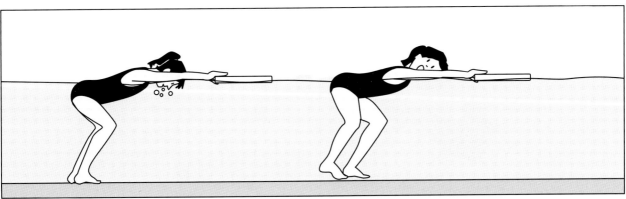

Practise breathing while walking across the pool

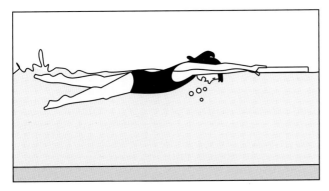

Practise breathing while kicking across the pool

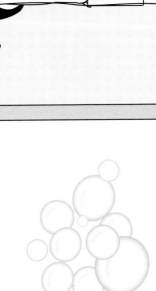

Drills for students

BODY ROTATION PRACTICE

The body should rotate on its long axis as it moves forward through the water.

The following practices are designed to teach students to rotate. These activities should not be attempted until students are streamlined and strong in their kicking. This will have developed from previous practices.

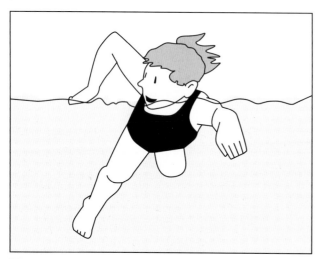

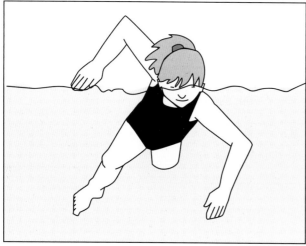

Freestyle body rotation drills highlighting high elbow recovery and bent arm pull

SIDE KICK PRACTICE

Students try freestyle kicking, lying on the side, one arm in front just below the surface, ear on that shoulder, other hand still by the side. They kick in a freestyle action sideways for a short distance (10–25 m). Students practise on alternate sides, changing at each end or side of the pool. During the kicking action, the knees should pass each other.

SIX–SIX PRACTICE

Students lie on the left side as above; after six kicks they rotate onto the right side, while making an underwater stroke with the left hand, exhaling as the face goes under and making a high elbow recovery with the right arm.

Any combination of less than six kicks can also be used (e.g. 3–3).

TIMING DRILLS
Catch-up stroke practice

The beginner holds one hand extended in front while the other arm completes a stroke, accompanied by continuous kicking of the legs. There is an endless number of patterns that may be used. A kickboard can be held out in front.

Some variations are:
- the same arm is used all the time
- left and right arms are used alternately
- three left and three right arm strokes are used alternately.

> **TEACHING TIP**
> The catch-up drill should not be used in excess. It is useful for students to develop the breathing timing. However, teachers should not allow them to become dependent on this drill to develop their swimming style.

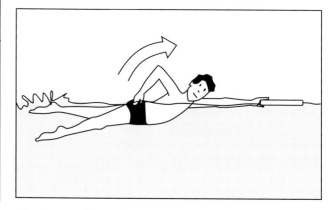

Catch-up stroke practice

Semi-catch-up stroke practice

In the semi-catch-up stroke practice, one hand is held extended in front until the recovery hand comes forward as far as the elbow of the front arm. Then the gliding hand commences an arm pull, while the other hand rests in the glide position.

Continuous kicking is important in the semi-catch-up timing. The arm strokes should be slowed down in front, so that there can be an acceleration as the hand moves through the underwater stroke.

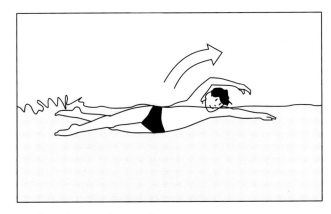

Semi catch-up stroke practice

Drills for advanced students

POWER STROKE PRACTICE

Power stroke is a continuous arm stroke style, for which the arms move almost opposite to each other. When one arm is in front, the other is at the back. At no time should both hands be seen in front of the head. A 6-, 4- or 2-beat kick rhythm may be used. Students should practise counting half the chosen number of kicks for each arm movement. Encourage students to practise short distances at first, with the face in for the whole distance. Later, they can practice over longer distances, adding breathing.

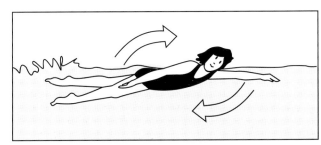

Advanced freestyle drill — power stroke practice

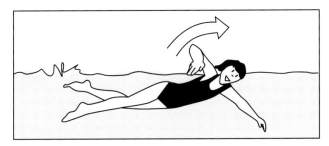

Advanced freestyle drill — high elbow

Progressions

The following steps support the initial teaching of freestyle with breathing in a regular pattern. Bilateral breathing may be introduced once the stroke has been learnt although some teachers wish to introduce bilateral breathing from the outset.

Catch-up drills are used to slow the stroke and allow students to concentrate on one arm, promote the development of a long stroke and avoid 'over-reaching' of the hands at entry.

Kickboards, when used in the progressions, are primarily intended to be a target for the hands and should be held at the back with the fingers over and the thumb under to promote the correct hand position on entry. These sequences assume a recovery at the end of each practice.

SUGGESTED STEPS

1. Glide and recovery

From a gliding position (shoulders under, arms forward):
- horizontal body position
- head submerged to the hairline
- exhaling in the water
- recovery to a standing position.

2. Glide with kick

From a gliding position:
- head submerged to the hairline
- horizontal body position
- exhaling in the water
- continuous kicking.

Kicking should be practised until it is effective in supporting a streamlined, horizontal body position.

3. Glide and kick with arm action

From a gliding position:
- glide and kick before adding the arm action
- exhaling in the water
- four or five strokes per repetition.

An alternating arm action without breathing is included at this stage to establish the whole skill.

4. Whole stroke

Alternating arm action:
- glide and kick before adding the arm action
- regular breathing on preferred side
- turning (not lifting) the head to breathe as required.

Return to starting from a gliding position once breathing is learned.

May introduce bilateral breathing now.

Bilateral breathing

- Combine bilateral breathing with arm action.
- Emphasise the rhythm ('1–2–breathe') with the entry of each arm.

Students accustomed to regular breathing may tend to exhale too completely prior to the second arm pull and may be assisted if they partially hold the breath during the early stage of the sequence.

Some teachers prefer to introduce bilateral breathing to a catch-up stroke, which may be promoted by the use of a board.

5. Refine the stroke

Continue refining the individual components of the stroke.

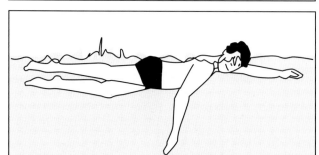

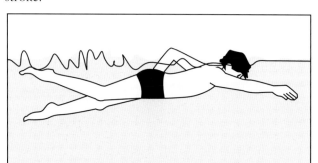

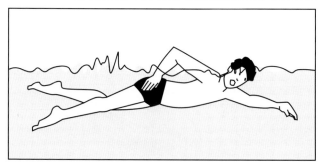

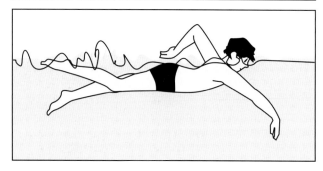

Freestyle sequence

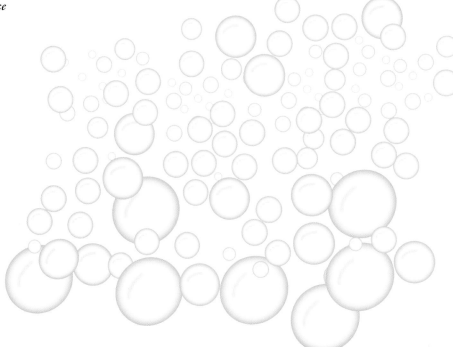

Evaluating technique

Look for the features listed below.

The overall timing, or flow, of the stroke is more important than the precision of each individual detail. Remember, an individual's success in freestyle depends on:

- smoothness as one arm takes over from the other, resulting in continuous propulsion
- 'high in the water' body position
- good body alignment, first on one side then the other
- balanced movements (right arm same as the left, same amount of bend, etc.)
- good head position (slightly raised at the forehead) and ease of breathing to either side
- efficient use of legs.

The following freestyle performance criteria have been identified as essential elements in an 'efficient' stroke development.

BODY POSITION

- During the stroke, check that the body rotates longitudinally on its side with one shoulder much higher than the other.
- Look for controlled body-tilting or rolling, with shoulders rolling the same amount to each side.
- Emphasise that shoulders are not held flat.

BASIC HEAD POSITION

- Look for an upward curve of the neck — the head lifted slightly so the waterline is about at the hairline.
- Emphasise that the head follows the body roll and remains in a comfortable, restful position. There should be no sudden lifts or turns of the head.

BREATHING

- Emphasise that breathing adds merely a few degrees of roll to the head, exposing the mouth to the air in the natural dip in the water. Note that this takes time to develop.
- Look for alternate side breathing — once every two or more strokes, in time with alternate arm entry. (This may be introduced later, after students have mastered single-sided breathing or breathing as required.)
- Emphasise that air is inhaled through the mouth and exhaled through the mouth and nose.
- Emphasise that the breath is *gently blown out*. Also, students *must not hold their breath* and need to be encouraged to exhale.

- The bilateral timing must be coordinated so that when the swimmer is breathing on the right side, the sequence commences immediately when the left hand enters the water; when breathing on the left side, the right hand entry triggers the breath.

LEG ACTION

- Continuous kicking action.
- Kick originates from hips.
- Legs are relaxed.
- Ankles are plantar-flexed (toes pointed) but loose.
- Legs are slightly bent on down-beat but straight on up-beat.

ARM ACTION

- Emphasise that hands are *not excessively cupped*, as it is preferable that fingers are held loosely together, creating a larger paddle. Have the student place their hand on their thigh and this should be the shape of the curved hand while swimming all strokes.
- For the arm entry, look for fingers entering first, followed by the wrist, the forearm and then the elbow. See that the thumb side of the hand is tilted slightly lower than the little-finger side.
- The hand should enter on the shoulder line. Emphasise that the arm pull starts slowly and gradually speeds up, with the arm looking as though it is curving downwards 'over a barrel'. In the middle of the pull, the elbows point to the side of the pool. The left hand makes a squashed 'S' and the right a reversed 'S' during the pull. See that the stroke ends prior to full extension, and that the thumb grazes the thigh as the hand moves into the recovery phase.
- Ensure that the hand does not cross the midline of the body.

RECOVERY

- For the recovery, watch that the shoulder appears first above the surface, followed by the upper arm, elbow, wrist and hand. See that the elbow is lifted high and the forearm swings around relatively loosely. The fingers then lead as the forearm is aimed to the re-entry point. This allows the forearm to be somewhat relaxed during this phase.
- Emphasise that the forearm and hand are completely relaxed through all but the final positioning, for the re-entry.

TIMING

- Note that it is the timing of the arm movements relative to each other that sets the two standard styles of freestyle apart.

- In the semi-catch-up freestyle stroke, emphasise that one arm moves through the last half of its pull, its entire recovery, then enters in front while the other arm moves through only the first half of the pull.
- In the power stroke freestyle, emphasise that there is little or no pause or glide of the hand in front. One arm enters barely in time to take over pulling before the other arm finishes the push.

The arm action is first introduced to students as a complete action (it is important not to over-analyse the skill at the point of introduction).

Students are encouraged to make large arm circles during the start of the arm action learning phase. As they gain confidence and skill, practices can be introduced to enable movement patterns of the 'technically correct' competitive stroke to be developed. Initial practices of the arm movement may take place on land prior to students entering the water. Following walking practice, the arm action can be developed with students in the prone gliding position. A kickboard may be used during the gliding practices when the arm action is being taught.

There is a school of thought that the technically correct arm action should be taught from the outset. However, most people believe that the technically correct action is far too complex a skill for students to master and the learning of the arm action through a sequence of practices is the preferred option.

Students often rush the arm action, usually because they do not feel confident lifting an arm out of the water. They must be reminded to practise continuous, slow strokes which take advantage of the body's natural buoyancy. This often needs to be reinforced every lesson, especially with young students.

Checklist for evaluating early beginner freestyle

- ❑ Relatively straight arms during pull and recovery phase.
- ❑ Continuous arm motion.
- ❑ Hands held relaxed.
- ❑ Breathing as required — promote extended breathing.
- ❑ Alternate-side (bilateral) breathing should be encouraged as skill improves.
- ❑ Continuous kicking.

Principles of movement in water for freestyle

RESISTANCE

The position of the body during freestyle should be as horizontal as possible — at or just below the surface of the water, depending on the body composition of the student. During elementary push and glide drills the depth of the head in the water should be adjusted to enable the heels of the feet to be at the surface of the water. Lifting the head will increase drag by 20–35 per cent.

The overall streamlined position enables frontal resistance to be minimised. The streamlining also serves to reduce eddy resistance. Frictional resistance cannot be effectively reduced and is therefore not considered.

The body, as viewed from above, should remain in a straight line. The rolling or swaying effect from the arm action should be minimised by ensuring that each hand does not cross the midline of the body and refraining from swinging arms wide to the side.

PROPULSION

The arms and hands provide the major propulsion in freestyle. Key considerations for efficient propulsion include:

1 The hand enters the water with minimal resistance — 'spearing the water'. It is usual for the thumb and index finger to enter first, followed by the wrist, forearm and elbow. During the entry the elbow is kept higher than the wrist.

2 Following the entry the hand slides forward and downwards until the arm straightens and the little finger begins to sweep outwards and downwards in a curvilinear path to 'catch' the water. The elbow gradually flexes to allow the palm of the hand to face backwards. The hand is now in a position to apply a force against the water and so propel the body forward. This action is related to the principle of 'propulsive drag'.

3 The insweep is the first propulsive phase of an arm stroke. The hand moves in a semi-circular motion to allow the hand and forearm to press firmly against still water. If the water begins to move backwards the application of force is significantly reduced.

4 The upsweep is the second and final phase of the arm stroke. It commences at the completion of the insweep and continues until the hand reaches the thigh. The elbow extends during the upsweep. During the insweep and upsweep the

hand accelerates and the hand pitches to push backwards against the water.

5 At the conclusion of the propulsive phase it is important that the hand leaves the water at the point where the hand releases pressure on the water to minimise resistance.

Legs and feet

The legs and feet provide a stabilising force and play a minor but important role in aiding propulsion. Of particular importance, however, is the impact the kicking action has on assisting the body in an almost horizontal and streamlined position. A flutter kick exceeding a depth of 30 cm causes frontal resistance, thus reducing speed. A deep kick may also affect the body position and cause eddies to form at the back of the legs.

To provide drive and propulsion from the kick, the toes must be pointed (or plantar-flexed) at the end of the down-beat. The water pressure forces the foot and ankle into plantar-flexion, if the ankle joint and surrounding muscles are relaxed. A pointed toe action minimises frontal resistance and allows the body to stabilise as it rotates on its horizontal axis.

Most of the kicking power originates from the hips, as they flex throughout the kicking action. Muscular force originates from the big thigh muscles, creating power for the down-beat. A flutter kick with an excessive knee bend slows down the swimmer, because no force is generated from the thigh muscles. A strong, efficient kick creates lift force, allowing the swimmer to 'ride' high in the water, minimising frontal resistance.

BREATHING

As the swimmer rotates on the horizontal axis, breathing is necessary for continuous stroking. The efficient swimmer creates a 'bow wave' in front of the head, allowing water to separate and rush off the body. The 'bow wave' produces air pockets on either side of the head, where the swimmer breathes. This gives the illusion that the swimmer is breathing underwater. As the swimmer rotates, the head rolls slightly to the side and air is inhaled.

The swimmer then turns the head to the centre of the body and gradually exhales. A head which is 'off centre' will cause frontal resistance. An excessive body roll, produced when inhaling air, causes deceleration and increases frontal resistance.

Summary

A successful freestyle stroke is dependent on efficient underwater sculling actions which provide approximately 80 per cent of the propulsion. The arm must be internally rotated (thumb down, palm facing outwards) to maximise propulsion and minimise injury. On hand entry, the hand/arm is sliced in the water to minimise turbulence and, on the hand exit, water is released by slicing the arm out. Effective sculling actions ensure that the body remains high in the water, minimising drag.

BACKSTROKE

Once students have developed confidence in gliding on the back in a streamlined position, the basics of backstroke can be taught.

Body position

To a large extent, the depth of the head determines the position of the body. For students, the ears should be just under the surface, eyes looking up at about a 70 degree angle and the body 'straight' and relaxed.

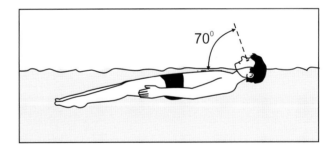

Backstroke body position

Leg action

Students must keep a continuous kick action going while learning the stroke. When practicing the kick, the toes should make a 'splash' on the surface, while the knees remain below.

The feet should not be too stiff, as ankle flexibility is very important. The toes should be turned naturally inwards and a low splash kick performed. The knees flex very slightly on the down-beat and straighten on the up-beat.

Kicking practices

Students may use a sculling action with the hands while initial kicking practices are being performed. Once reasonable propulsion is being obtained a kickboard may be held to practice the action.

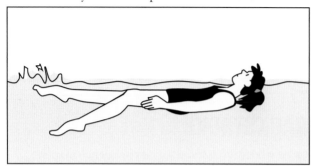

Backstroke kicking

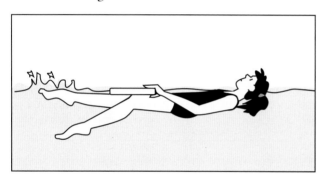

Backstroke kick, holding board over knees to promote correct action

Arm action

TEACHING TIP

The whole-skill teaching method is again the best method to introduce the arm stroke and only if students are experiencing difficulty should the skill be taught in individual parts.

While performing the arm stroke, the body should not be rigid in the water but rotate smoothly from side to side to assist the entry and recovery of the hands and arms.

The entry into the water is made by the back of the hand or little-finger first (palm outwards) at an 11 o'clock right-hand and a 1 o'clock left-hand position.

The entry should be smooth, with a minimal amount of turbulence being created. It is important that students do not over-reach to keep the body in a streamlined position. Following entry, the arm remains straight and sweeps downwards and outwards to a depth of approximately 40 cm. This varies with the size of the learner.

Also, immediately following the entry, the hand rotates to be facing slightly downwards from the vertical as the elbow begins to flex and pressure is applied to the palm of the hand. The ability to catch the water is considered to be the most important aspect of the stroke.

The elbow continues to flex until it is bent to approximately a 90 degree angle at the end of the pulling action and the forearm rotates so the fingertips are relatively close to the surface of the water.

During this upward, backward and inward movement the hand should begin to accelerate.

Once the shoulder is level with the hand the palm begins a downward and outward movement until the hip passes the hand. The palm finishes the propulsive phase by facing the bottom of the pool.

The shoulder lifts, followed by the arm and then the hand. The back of the hand of the recovery arm is uppermost as the hand leaves the water. When the recovery arm reaches the vertical position, the palm faces outwards, slightly ready for a smooth, turbulence-free re-entry with the hand entering little-finger first.

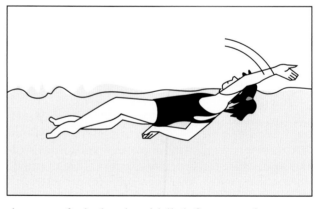

Arm entry for backstroke, with little finger entering water first

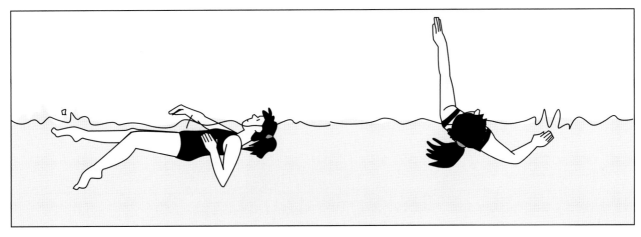

Backstroke arm pull, demonstrating bent arm pull to maximise efficiency

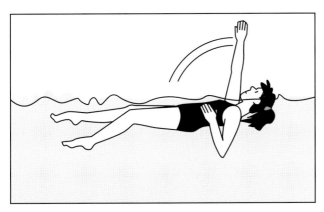

Backstroke push phase, highlighting the final push to gain maximum distance per stroke

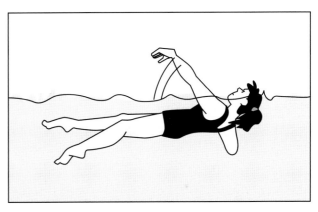

Arm recovery of backstroke, demonstrating a relaxed and extended arm

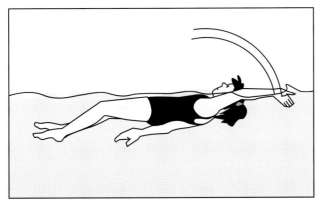

Recovery arm enters the water first, as opposite arm completes propulsive phase

BREATHING

While initial kicking practices are being performed, students should be encouraged to breathe as naturally as possible and to avoid holding the breath.

Drills for students

ARM PRACTICES

One-arm practice

Students swim using one arm only over the practice distance. The hand should be rotated during the recovery so that the little finger enters first, palm facing outwards. They continue until the hand is at a depth of up to 40 cm.

Allow students to complete the underwater stroke without further direction at this time. Remember that the objective of the one-arm drill at this stage is to make the link between recovery, entry and catch.

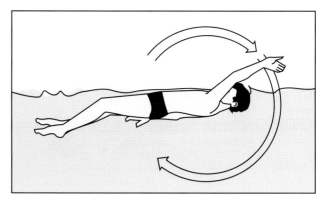

Backstroke one-arm practice

PROPULSION PRACTICES

Lane-rope practice

Students swim, using one arm only, alongside a lane rope (or handrail), grasping the rope with an under-grip to pull and push the body along. This practice aims to develop the desirable arm movement of bending and then straightening in the underwater stroke.

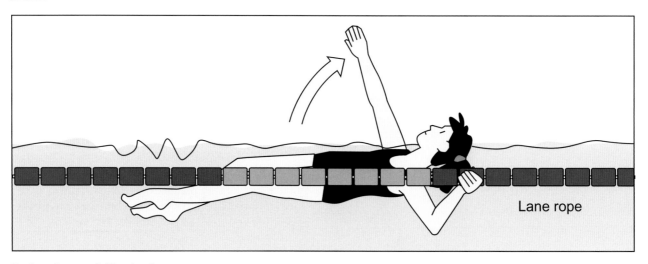

Backstroke arm drill using lane rope

Drills for advanced students

ARM-RECOVERY PRACTICES

The periscope practice

With one hand held by the side (palm down), the other arm is raised to a near vertical position, with the wrist relaxed and the back of the hand uppermost. Good body position is maintained, and strong kicks over a given practice distance (10–25 m).

Changing periscope practice

Raise and lower the arms alternately through 90 degrees to a count of 'right–2–3–left–2–3'.

    The periscope practices are designed to develop a vertical movement pattern in the recovery, with the arm reaching up and straight except for a relaxed wrist.

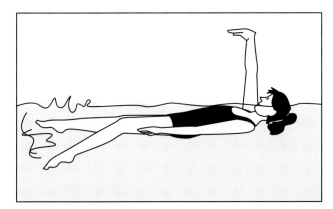

The periscope practice

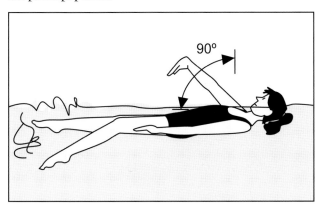

Periscope practice — let the water drip off your fingers

ROTATION/STREAMLINING PRACTICES

As students progress they should begin to rotate more on the long axis of the body. This can then be attempted with the body rotating to approximately 70 degrees past the horizontal on each side.

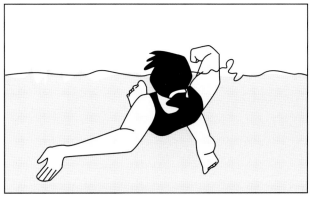

Body rotation on the long axis

TIMING ARM ACTION AND BREATHING

Once students have acquired a sound arm technique, emphasis may be given to the timing of the arm action to the breathing. As one hand enters, students take a breath and, while the opposite hand enters, they exhale.

TIMING/STREAMLINING PRACTICES

Gliding backstroke — six count

Students hold one arm extended in front and one arm by the side for a count of six kicks, then change position of the arms, with one recovering and entering while the other performs the three sweeps under the water:

    'Hold–2–3–4–5–6, change O–V–E–R.'

Check:

- body position
- a smooth changeover
- kicking technique
- correct arm movement patterns.

Gliding backstroke — three count

Students repeat above, to the following count:

    'Hold–2–3, change O–V–E–R.'

Measured backstroke

Evenness of stroke rhythm is the key factor in successful and economic backstroke. Students should 'measure out' the strokes by counting 1–2–3 for each arm where '1' coincides with the entry of the hand.

Progressions

SUGGESTED STEPS

1. Glide and recovery

From a gliding position (shoulders under, head back):

- horizontal body position
- head submerged to the crown
- chin slightly tucked in; recovery to a standing position.

It is preferable to teach the recovery first.

2. Glide and kick

- Horizontal body position.
- Head submerged to the crown.
- Chin slightly tucked in.
- Continuous kick without excessive knee bend.

Kicking should be practiced until it is effective in supporting a streamlined, horizontal body position.

Option

Repeat with arms extended behind head in a streamlined position.

The ability to glide and kick with the arms extended back will greatly improve body position and should be progressively developed, receiving additional attention during the following steps.

3. Glide with kick and arm action

With and without the use of a kickboard:

- horizontal body position; board held over thighs (fingers on top)
- simple continuous arm action.

Drills with a catch-up to the thigh may become habitual and should be interspersed with practice of an alternating arm action.

4. Whole stroke

Alternating arm action:

- horizontal body position
- simple arm action as above.

5. Breathing

Breathe in on one arm and breathe out on the other.

6. Refine the stroke

Continue refining the individual components of the stroke.

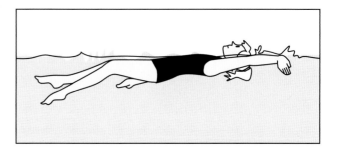
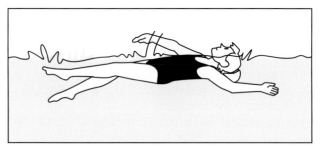
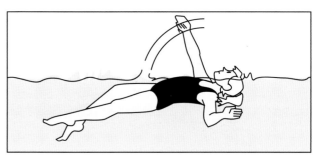
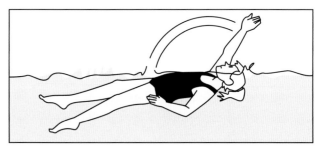
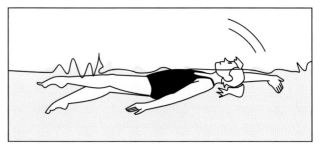

Backstroke sequence

Evaluating technique

Teachers should look for the features listed below. The overall timing, or flow, of the stroke is more important than the precision of details.

Remember, success in backstroke depends on:

- smoothness as one arm takes over from the other
- a high body position in the water
- balanced movements (right arm is a mirror image of the left)
- maintaining a comfortable but steady head position
- a steady, consistent kick
- pulling, using the bent arm pull-and-push action.

The following backstroke performance criteria have been identified as essential elements of an efficient stroke.

BODY AND HEAD POSITIONS

- The body is slightly curved with the hips lower than the head and feet.
- The pulling shoulder should sink down almost under the neck.
- Emphasise that there is a slight bend of the body-line at the hips. See that the hips are submerged slightly, but not in a sitting position.
- Make sure the beginner's chest is at the surface. When at high speed, emphasise that the torso, from the waist up, is above the surface.
- See that the chin is *not* pressed against the chest or tilted back to see forward.
- The ears should be just under the surface, eyes looking up at about a 70 degree angle and the body 'straight' and relaxed.

LEG ACTION

- Watch for a steady, continuous kick. It is essential in good backstroke swimming. See that the kick has a moderate bend of the knees (about 30 degrees) and the knees are *not* breaking the surface. See that the direction of the kick is forcing water 'backwards'.

ARM ACTION

- For the arm entry, see that the little-finger side of the hand enters first.
- For the recovery, emphasise that at the end of the pull, the arm lifts out of the water straight and moves over the shoulder (not with thumb first). As the arm lifts, so does the shoulder, as if to lift the arm even higher.
- For the pull, see that the hand and arm pass through the surface, down to a depth of approximately 40 cm to catch the water. As the elbow flexes, the palm presses against the water as it moves upwards towards the surface. Emphasise that the arm bend increases as the pull continues and that midway through the pull the elbow points to the bottom of the pool as the arm bends 90 degrees. Finally, see that the hand pushes downwards as the arm slowly straightens through the second half of the stroke. Make sure the push ends with a vigorous downwards throwing action. This is called the 'push phase' in backstroke.

BREATHING

- Watch for a regular breathing pattern, preferably breathing in on one arm and out on the other.

TIMING

Emphasise that the arms are not opposite to each other in timing. The recovery arm speeds up as it moves to enter well before the pulling arm finishes the underwater phase of the arm stroke.

Checklist for evaluating beginner backstroke

- ❑ Head back, chest up, streamlined position.
- ❑ Continuous kicking and smooth arm action.
- ❑ Breathing naturally (ideally breathing in on the recovery of one arm and out on the recovery of the other arm).
- ❑ Arm recovery commencing with the back of hand leaving the water.
- ❑ Relatively straight arms during the recovery phase.
- ❑ Down–up–down propulsive arm action.
- ❑ Body rotates on long axis but head remains still.

Principles of movement in water for backstroke

RESISTANCE

The backstroke body position must be as horizontal as possible, streamlined and close to the water's surface. Like freestyle, backstroke relies on the propulsion of the arms and hands for optimal movement. The flutter kick used in backstroke also acts as a stabilising force, but the up-beat provides the drive — the reverse effect of freestyle.

An inclined body position creates frontal resistance and turbulence, due to an inefficient kick and, possibly, a fear of not being able to see the direction of travel. Successful backstroke depends on a fluent body roll to maximise the power of the upper body, and a fast flutter kick to create speed and balance.

Frontal resistance is produced if the body is not horizontal and the kick is too deep; that is, exceeding a depth of 30 cm. Wide, sweeping arm actions also cause resistance and turbulence.

Effective sculling movements minimise turbulence and frontal resistance. Lift force is a product of sculling, to allow positive forward movement, and an elevated body position, to reduce drag.

PROPULSION

Key considerations for efficient backstroke include the following:

1 A carefully executed hand entry is important at the start of the underwater pull–push phase. The little finger enters the water first as the arm is outstretched in the 11 o'clock position (right hand). A careful entry ensures that turbulence is reduced. Air bubbles are created around the body if the hand 'crashes' down on the water, rather than making a 'sliced and streamlined' entry. Eddy turbulence is minimised if the hand enters with control.

2 As the hand starts the catchphase, the wrist must be firm to effectively 'grip' onto the water. A good catch ensures the body is gaining significant movement. A floppy wrist is ineffective as the swimmer loses speed at the most critical part of the stroke. The hand should travel to a depth no greater than 40 cm and begin the catch and pull phases. A good catch depth ensures the pull and push is maximised, allowing for the 90 degree arm bend to produce optimal power.

3 As the hand travels through the pull phase, the elbow is bent at 90 degrees in line with the shoulder. At this point the arm will form a 'V' shape to increase arm power. The body's leverage system — the arms and legs — works to gain maximum power by producing the greatest muscular force. Angling the arms and legs effectively increases stroke efficiency.

4 The push is a downward sweep to the thigh, with the palm of the hand facing the bottom of the pool. A long stroke ensures the body's propulsive forces are effective, by gaining the greatest distance per stroke. The downward sweep creates lift force, elevating the body to ride on the water's surface. As the hand pushes against the water, it travels backwards and downwards. The opposite then occurs — the body travels forward and upwards. Gravity acts to stabilise the body at the water's surface.

LEGS AND FEET

The legs and feet play a crucial role in backstroke by supporting the body as the torso rotates to gain optimal power and speed. The up-beat of the backstroke kick provides the most drive as the thigh muscles contract to create force.

Plantar-flexion of the feet ensures that movement will be efficient. The feet also angle in towards the body's midline — a movement called 'inversion'. The forces of the water allow inversion to occur naturally, if the surrounding muscles are relaxed.

Summary

Efficient backstroke requires various practice drills to enhance fluency and increase stroke rate.

The arm and hand speed during the underwater phase is crucial, so that maximum distance per stroke is achieved while maintaining a high stroke rate. A fluent body rotation produces maximum force from the big muscles of the upper body and is complemented by the additional drive of the strong flutter kick.

BREASTSTROKE

Following the development of the basic learner sequence, attention can be directed to the teaching of breaststroke. Breaststroke is an important stroke to teach beginner swimmers because of its survival values. It is also one of the four competitive strokes and has a certain quality which gives swimmers a great deal of pleasure when performing it.

The advantages of the stroke from a survival perspective are that:

- the limbs recover under the water
- a rest or glide phase can be developed to conserve energy
- the head may be kept clear of the water to allow for a natural breathing style
- a clear view to the front is obtained.

When teaching breaststroke, students should be encouraged to practice appropriate movement patterns to develop symmetrical limb movements. Symmetrical movements conform to the competitive rules of the stroke but, more importantly, maximise the propulsive effect.

Body position

Students should stand with the feet beside each other and slightly apart, the knees bent to allow the shoulders to be under the water. The arms extend forward in front of the shoulders and the chin rests on the water.

Following a normal breath, the face is placed into the water until approximately one-third of the head is in the water with the face looking forward and downward. Students push off smoothly to glide. During the glide phase the shoulders, buttocks and heels are at the surface of the water with the toes extended in a streamlined position. Adjustments to the head position may be made if the heels do not remain just under surface.

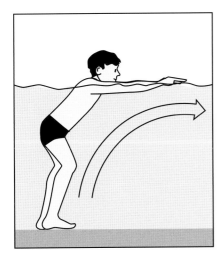

Starting position for breaststroke at the beginner level, before commencing the glide

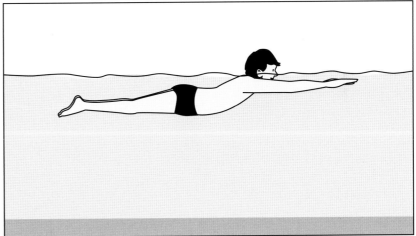

Breaststroke push and glide

Leg action

The kick requires the legs to move simultaneously and in the same horizontal plane.

Students should be given a brief introduction to the actual kicking technique during out-of-water practices. They should lie on a bench or the edge of the pool with the legs extended. The knees bend to draw the heels towards the buttocks. When the knees are fully flexed, the feet rotate into the 'hooked' and 'V' position, ready for the propulsive part of the kick. When students perform the movement efficiently, practice in water can commence.

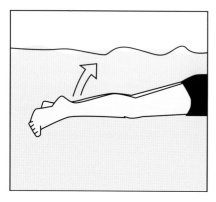 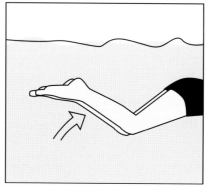 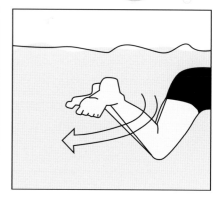

Breaststroke leg and feet actions during recovery and propulsive phases

When in water, students should stand about waist-deep, with the feet apart and level with each other. They should bend the knees to allow the shoulders to be under the water. Arms should be stretched forward, shoulder-width apart, with the palms facing the bottom of the water. On a signal, students place the face in the water with the head a little deeper than the hairline and push off into a gliding position. During the glide, the feet should assume the inverted dorsi-flexed 'V' position. When the glide is performed well, the kicking action can be introduced. The phases of the kicking action should be:

> push off, glide, kick, glide, stand with feet together.

When one kick can be performed correctly, a sequence of kicks can be linked together:

> push off, glide, kick, glide, kick, glide, stand with feet together.

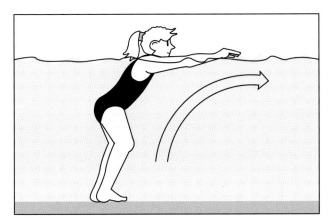
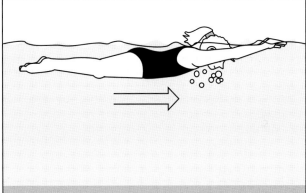
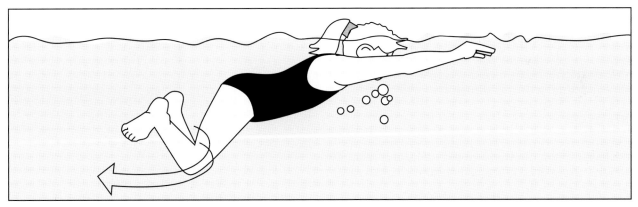
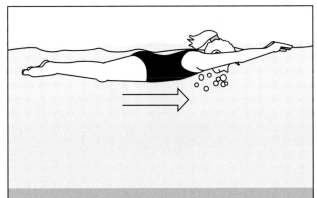
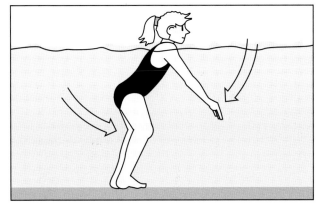

Breaststroke sequence — push off, glide, kick, glide, stand with feet together

Once a sequence of kicks can be performed satisfactorily, the breathing technique can be introduced.

Arm action

It is important that the arms move simultaneously and that there is no pushing phase, except during the start and at the turns. The arm action may be divided into three distinct segments:

- catch and outsweep
- downsweep and insweep
- recovery.

CATCH AND OUTSWEEP

The arm action commences with the arms fully extended, hands close together up to 20 cm below the surface with the palms turned outwards. The initial movement of the arms is a push outwards until the hands are wider than the shoulders. During this phase of the stroke, the palms of the hands should be applying considerable force on the water. Students should be encouraged to keep the elbows locked straight during this phase to enhance the likelihood of symmetrical movements.

DOWNSWEEP AND INSWEEP

The lower arms and wrists rotate inwards to enable the palms to face towards the feet as the arms press against the water, while the elbows remain high. When the palms come to a position below the elbows, they sweep inwards to complete the propulsive phase of the stroke. The hands do not pass back beyond the shoulders during the arm stroke.

RECOVERY

Once the pressure on the water has been released from the palms of the hands, the elbows and hands squeeze towards the midline of the body before extending to a fully stretched position, palms facing downwards.

As the arms reach full extension, they are pressed down to 20 cm, ready for the commencement of the next stroke. This action keeps the hips from dropping and consequently assists with the maintenance of a streamlined body position.

Students do not seem to have a great deal of difficulty in learning the arm action. Students can gain initial understanding of the arm action by drawing circular patterns with the hands and arms. If the circular patterns are practised in the water, students should stand with one foot in front of the other to provide support and have the shoulders below the surface.

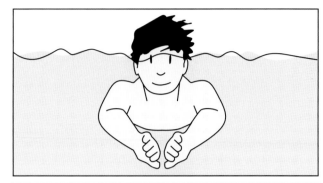

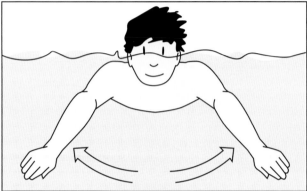

Breaststroke catch and outsweep

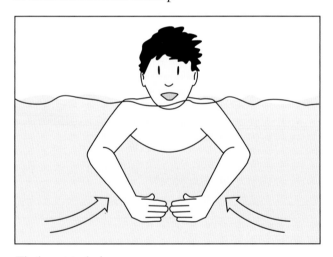

The breaststroke insweep

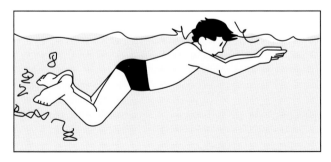

Breaststroke leg propulsion and arm recovery

Breathing technique

As in any swimming stroke, breathing should be as natural as possible. A natural breathing technique implies that swimmers neither hyperventilate nor hold the breath for an extended period of time.

Initial breathing practice should include students lowering the face into the water and exhaling through both the mouth and nose while standing.

The next stage is to hold a kickboard with the hands apart at the back of the board, fingers on top, thumbs underneath and the arms extended. The kick should be performed with the chin on the water and eyes looking forward. This practice can be repeated, but with the face in the water and with exhalation. The face should come clear of the water with the chin touching the water to inhale through the mouth. The face must remain in the water until the kick is completed. When the heels come together, the head should be raised to take a fresh breath.

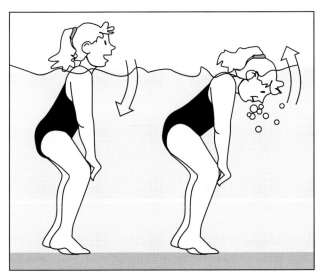

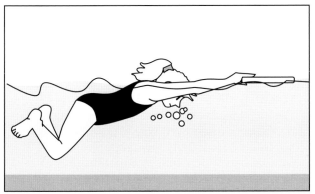

Breaststroke breathing practice

Coordination of the stroke

The coordination of the breaststroke action varies according to whether the stroke is being performed for survival or for competitive purposes.

Survival breaststroke has a significant glide or resting phase, the purpose of which is to conserve energy. Additionally, it has a slower relative hand and foot speed throughout the stroke.

Competitive breaststroke also has a glide phase, but the speed of the hands and feet is significantly faster, and therefore the glide is shorter. To obtain an efficient breaststroke technique, it is imperative that the body does not bob up and down as a result of incorrect timing of the leg and arm actions. The correct timing of the stroke occurs when the kick is completed and the arms are fully extended with the body streamlined in the water. At the conclusion of each stroke, whether for survival or competition, the hands-together, legs-together (i.e. streamlined) position must be obtained.

COMBINING KICK AND ARM STROKE

The ultimate sequence is to push from a wall or standing position, followed by a glide then pull–breathe–kick–glide sequence, with the glide being extended for between 1 and 3 seconds. Following the push from the wall, students should complete an arm stroke and during the stroke lift the head for a breath. This practice may be followed by a further sequence of kick–glide–pull–breathe, which repeats and continues.

Students feel comfortable with this sequence, and once it has been developed, it does not require relearning or extensive modification — just refinement. Breaststroke, when performed correctly, provides students with a relaxed and efficient stroke that can be used in a variety of different aquatic situations.

Drills for students

KICKING PRACTICES

- With a kickboard, students place hands apart at the back of the board, fingers on top, thumbs underneath and arms extended. They work on symmetry, ankles flexing and feet turning out on recovery.
- With a kickboard, students place the face in water after a 'normal' breath, push off and glide then kick and glide and raise the head to the front to breathe after exhaling.
- Without a kickboard, students have arms extended and shoulder-width apart. They push off and glide, then kick and glide, exhale, raise the head and breathe. They practice a sequence of kicks.

WHOLE-STROKE PRACTICES

Kick–kick–pull

The aim of kick–kick–pull is that students should develop the feeling of driving the body forward over the hands. The legs should remain together and straight until the *insweep* of the arms is complete and the legs kick as the arms are stretching in front, with the head between them.

Kick–pull

The aim of kick–pull is that students should improve whole-stroke timing. The arms sweep while the legs glide, and the legs and arms recover as the body moves forward from the propulsion provided by the arms and previous kicks. The legs sweep before the speed of the body decreases and while the head and arms are streamlined in the front.

Drills for advanced students

KICKING

With hands trailing behind by the hips, students raise the heels on recovery to touch the hands, outsweep, downsweep, insweep, ankles stretch, glide. Students should aim to develop length in the movement pattern and maintain the timing of breathing, leg sweeps and glides.

GLIDING KICK

Students count the number of leg movements required to cover a given distance (e.g. 25 m). 'Breathe, leg sweep, glide'. They start the next movement as the body begins to slow down. Ten is a good number for 25 m.

ARM PRACTICES

Pulling

- With a pull-buoy between the legs and the face in the water, students practice the arm movement pattern.

Pulling and breathing

- Perform as above, with exhalation on *recovery* and inhalation on *downsweep*.
- With a pull-buoy between the legs and breathing on each stroke. Left arm–right arm.

WHOLE-STROKE PRACTICES

The following practices aim to develop a dolphin-like movement:

- students swim one double-arm stroke and breaststroke kick, followed by two dolphin kicks
- students swim one double-arm stroke and breaststroke kick, followed by one dolphin kick
- students swim one double-arm stroke and breaststroke kick, allowing the legs to rise on their glide as though preparing to perform the down-beat of the dolphin kick. The trunk and head should come up and forward on the *downsweep* of the arms. Teachers should note, this style will not suit everyone.

Progressions

The leg actions for survival backstroke and breaststroke are similar. They differ only with regard to the degree of hip-flexion employed, with survival backstroke using slightly less.

TEACHING TIP
The initial teaching of breaststroke leg action on the back has proved very effective and is suggested below. Thus the development of survival backstroke prior to breaststroke is a possible option. Steps for developing the leg actions for both strokes are similar.

SUGGESTED STEPS

1. Foot exercises

Sitting, with legs extended:

- toes point down
- feet turn out (dorsi-flexed).

2. Leg action sitting

On edge of pool or similar:

- thighs unsupported, leaning backwards slightly
- knees slightly apart
- limited hip-flexion
- feet move outside line of knees in circling action.

Use passive manipulation to direct movement:

- students push against teacher's hands (pressure on inside of foot)
- avoid pulling legs through movement.

3. Backward glide and recovery

From a gliding position (shoulders underwater, head leaning back):

- horizontal body position
- head submerged to the crown
- chin slightly tucked in; recovery to a standing position.

Teach the recovery first.

4. Leg action on back

From a gliding position (with board or sculling):

- glide, single kick, glide initially
- number of kicks gradually increasing
- toes turn out before kick
- shoulders, hips and knees horizontal
- limited hip-flexion
- glide between kicks.

Option

Introduce survival backstroke arm action and coordination.

See survival backstroke progressions (on page 168).

5. Leg action lying on front

While lying:

- half in, top half raised out of water
- supported by arms on edge
- toes turned out before kick
- shoulders, hips and knees level
- pause between kicks.

6. Glide with kick on front

From a gliding position:

- glide, single kick plus glide initially
- arms extended forward (to board)
- number of kicks gradually increasing
- glide between kicks.

Exhaling in the water may be included. This will improve body position and assist students whose legs sink rapidly.

7. Glide with kick and breathing

From a gliding position:

- glide with limited number of kicks initially
- inhaling during recovery of the legs
- exhaling during the kick and glide
- whole of face submerged for exhalation.

8. Arm action

a. Shoulders over lane rope or a noodle, or
b. lying with shoulders over pool edge:

- hands press outwards
- hands scull inwards below the chin
- elbows high until the end of the inward scull
- pause for the glide phase.

With breathing:

- inhaling during the inward scull
- exhaling during forward extension and glide.

9. Coordination of whole stroke

One complete stroke

From a gliding position:

- glide before commencing the stroke
- standing after each stroke
- significant glide with arms extended
- exhaling during the glide
- reinforce the kick–glide–pull–breathe sequence.

When the water is more than waist-deep push off from the pool side in place of the first kick. If the pool side is used, students should ensure that the glide is gentle or the propulsive effect of the hands will be lost, the arms may pull too far back and coordination will suffer.

Consecutive strokes

The number of strokes should be progressively increased according to success as long as symmetry and coordination can be maintained.

Holding the glide phase for a three-count will assist with promoting the desired timing.

10. Refine the stroke

Continue refining the individual components of the stroke.

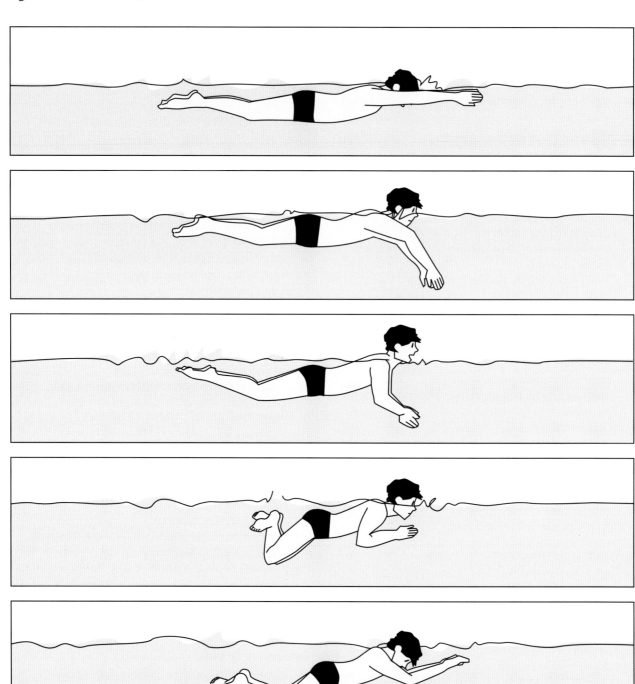

Breaststroke sequence

Evaluating technique

The overall timing, or flow, of the stroke is more important than precision of the details. Remember, the stroke resembles a series of gentle lifts and lunges forward. The following breaststroke descriptions have been identified as essential elements in an efficient stroke.

BODY POSITION

The sequence of the stroke is important and the kick–glide–pull–breathe sequence should be consistent.

HEAD POSITION

- Make sure the head is held relaxed and steady, riding up and down with the shoulders.
- There should be no separate lifting or bobbing motions of the head.

LEG ACTION

- See that the knees are separated no wider than shoulder-width.
- See that the kick is started by rotating the toes outwards and flexing them towards the shins in a swift, deliberate action. As the feet are swept into the propulsive phase, see that the push action is led by the knees.

ARM ACTION

- In the arm action, watch that when the arms are extended in front they are aimed downwards with about 20 cm of water above the hands.
- See that the pull starts with the hands tilted thumb-side down and the palms facing outwards. The wrists flex first and the arms move slowly apart, with the forearms descending and the upper arms remaining high. The arms sweep outwards until the elbows are in line with the forehead. Then the hands sweep swiftly inwards, followed by the elbows. With that, the final thrust of the hands and forearms is vigorous and aimed slightly downwards, with the elbows about 15 or 20 cm apart. The arm action should not be too wide.
- Watch for an inverted heart shape scribed by the hands during the pull. See that the arm action is continuous, quickening as it progresses. There should be no hesitation while inhaling.

BREATHING

Look for inhalation on every stroke when the shoulders rise, lifting the face clear of the water, as the hands complete the pull phase just prior to recovery. Exhale through mouth and nose, into the water — during the pull phase.

 ## Checklist for evaluating beginner breaststroke

- ☐ Body as streamlined as possible to reduce resistance.
- ☐ Symmetrical limb movements.
- ☐ Leg kick in the same horizontal plane.
- ☐ When the knees are fully flexed, the feet rotate into the 'dorsi-flexed' position.
- ☐ Arms move simultaneously through the pull after the glide.
- ☐ Hands do not push back past the shoulders.
- ☐ Glide action always follows the kick.
- ☐ Breathing is as natural as possible.

Principles of movement in water for breaststroke

RESISTANCE

Breaststroke is the slowest competitive stroke because the arm recovery and leg recovery create frontal resistance. The underwater actions of the arms and legs cause water to hit the thighs and arms, resulting in deceleration. The high degree of resistance created in breaststroke has resulted in dramatic changes to the stroke at the highest competitive levels. The 'wave-style' breaststroke produces an undulating action so that the body is riding high on the water. The dolphin-like action allows the swimmer to be elevated and minimises frontal resistance.

The glide phase is important in elementary skill practices so that the timing of the stroke is emphasised. This helps to minimise turbulence because the body is streamlined. The feet must come together at the end of the kick to promote a streamlined body position. It is common for swimmers to continue onto the next stroke cycle without completing the propulsive phase properly. The hands-together, feet-together positions should be attained before the propulsive phase is completed.

Eddy turbulence is also a problem when the heels move towards the buttocks in the leg recovery, creating swirls of disturbed water and slowing down the swimmer. A high body position and good knee-flexion minimise both eddy and frontal resistance. The face should be in the water as the arms complete the recovery, so that the streamlined effect is maximised. An elevated head during the recovery creates an inclined body position, thus increasing frontal resistance. The head carefully extends forward as the arms start the recovery.

PROPULSION

Key considerations for efficient breaststroke include the following:

1 The catch of the breaststroke arm action is important to maximise the propulsive forces of the arms and upper body. The wrists must be firm and palms face backwards and downwards as the catch starts. The hands sweep out wider than the shoulders in a sculling action. When the hand 'grips' onto the water, propulsive drag is produced, as the hand creates an axis point for the body to pass over when the arm lengthens.

2 The insweep of the arm action provides the greatest amount of lift in the stroke, allowing the upper body to rise. The shoulders come out of the water and the body is inclined. At this point air is inhaled. A breath is always taken at the point that maximum lift is produced. This minimises frontal resistance and ensures that coordination of the stroke is maintained.

3 During the insweep of the arms, the movement is accelerated using a sculling action. This maximises forward propulsion and lift. The legs also accelerate during the propulsive phase to create a 'whipping' action. The accelerated movements produce maximum power, because the speed at which the muscles contract is increased. Continuous accelerated sculling actions produce constant forward movement.

4 The arm and leg recovery is usually slower than the powerful propulsive phases. They actually increase frontal resistance and create eddy turbulence around the feet and legs. The feet should be loosely pointed during recovery to conserve energy.

   Dorsi-flexion also places the feet in the correct position to grip onto the water in the propulsive phase. The inside of the foot and lower leg or calf catches the water and the body travels forward as the legs straighten.

5 In the arm recovery, the hands meet together under the chin but they may be angled in an open or closed position — like an open book or a hands-in-prayer position. Swimmers have achieved success with both methods, although the open-hand angle is better suited to the wave-style technique because the hands do not create significant frontal resistance in the recovery. The teacher should encourage the method which suits the individual, depending on the efficiency of the sculling actions. The traditional closed-hand position may be better suited to students.

Summary

Breaststroke creates a considerable amount of drag, which has been successfully minimised by coaches who strive to find a faster alternative. Because leg and arm recovery occur under the water, the speed of breaststroke will not significantly change. The stroke has evolved into a stroke which is close to the water's surface and is constantly undulating to create the dolphin-like action.

BUTTERFLY

Following the acquisition of the basic learner sequence of skills, components of butterfly can be taught. Butterfly is often taught later in the student's stroke development as it is perceived to be difficult to master. This is not necessarily the case and elementary practices of the basic butterfly stroke skills may be introduced earlier than is often the current practice. The learning of butterfly provides a challenge to beginner students and many gain a high degree of personal reward from performing the stroke efficiently. The sequence for introducing butterfly is similar to that for the other strokes, with the kick being developed following the performance of a streamlined gliding position.

Body position

The body position is a streamlined prone position; the leg action provides an undulating motion for the torso.

Leg action

The butterfly kick is often referred to as a dolphin kick and is a powerful action which often provides students with a great deal of satisfaction. During the kicking action, the legs are close together and move simultaneously.

   The kicking action consists of a down-beat and an up-beat performed in a continuous manner. The down-beat commences with the knees bent and the ankles just out of the water. The feet should be pointed and turned in slightly (pigeon-toed). During the down-beat, the legs are forcefully extended or straightened, resulting in a lifting of the hips. On the up-beat the knees bend and the hips go down. Throughout the kicking action it is important for students to maintain an undulating body position. The kick must be initiated from the hips and involves the entire body when performed successfully.

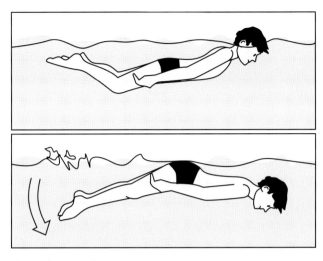

Butterfly leg action

KICKING PRACTICES

The following kicking practices are useful for students:

'The Man from Atlantis' or 'Aquaman'

- Students submerge, push off from the side, extend the arms in front and dolphin kick along the bottom of the shallow end for a short distance.
- Encourage flexibility of hip, knee and ankle joints.

Dolphin kick on back

- Students lie in the back-glide position, with hands trailing in the water.
- The students dolphin kick, feeling the hips bend and straighten and the water push up from the feet.

Dolphin torpedo

Dolphin torpedo is performed:
- with arms extended in front
- with hands on hips.

Dolphin kick with kickboard

When practising the dolphin kick with kickboard:
- emphasis is on the first beat
- emphasis is then on the second beat.

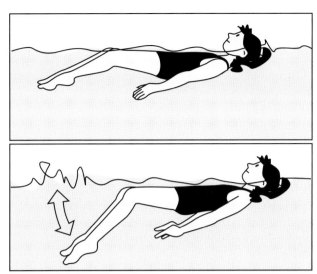

Dolphin kick on back

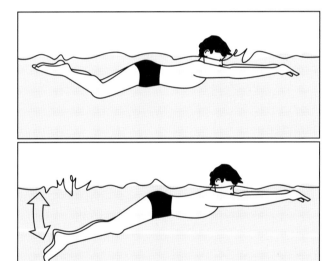

Dolphin torpedo

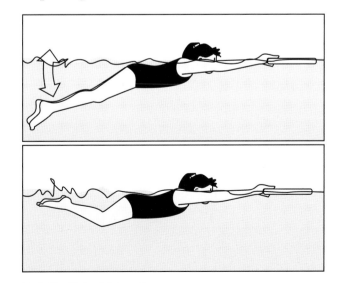

Dolphin kick with board

Arm action

The butterfly stroke is often considered to be the most difficult of the competitive strokes to perform because the arms recover over the water at the same time. Before teaching the butterfly arm action, it is necessary to have a sound understanding of the fundamentals involved.

ENTRY AND CATCH

The hands enter the water at shoulder width, with the palms facing outwards to allow the hands to slide smoothly into the water. The hands should submerge up to about 20 cm below the surface of the water. After entry:

- the hands sweep outwards until they are wider than the shoulders
- the palms slowly rotate in towards the end of the outsweep until they face back.

The entry is a gentle movement and little propulsion occurs. During the catch, the hands accelerate and provide propulsive force.

The purpose of the catch is to 'set the scene' for the propulsive insweep.

INSWEEP

The insweep is the first of the two most propulsive phases of the stroke. During the insweep:

- the arms sweep downwards, inwards and then upwards in a semicircular movement until they are under the shoulders, close to the midline of the body

- the hands should be pitched to allow the water to be deflected backwards over the palms from the thumb to the little-finger side
- the hand speed accelerates.

UPSWEEP

The upsweep is the second of the major propulsive phases of the stroke. The upsweep commences as the hands come close together under the midline of the body. During the upsweep the hand direction changes to a backward, outward and upward movement until the hands come close to the surface, beside the thighs, ready for the release.

The upsweep is usually the most powerful and propulsive part of the stroke.

ARM RECOVERY

The release of the hands occurs just prior to the arms fully extending and before the hands reach the surface.

- The release is made by turning the palms of the hands inwards to allow the hands to be slid from the water with a minimum of resistance.
- The arms must be extended during the exit from the water to allow a circling up, out and forward movement to occur.
- The arms and hands skim above the surface of the water until the entry is made.
- During the over-water recovery, the palms of the hands should face inwards during the first half and be rotated outwards during the second half. The head is lowered with the chin pressed towards the neck.

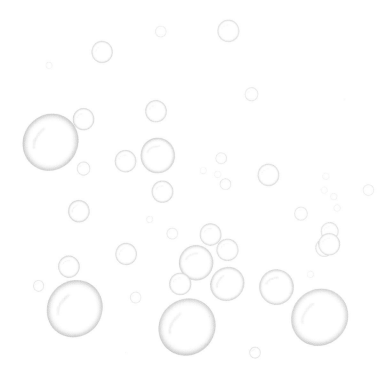

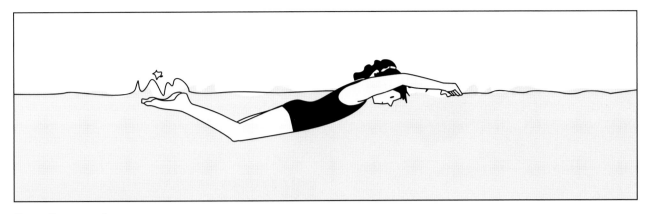

Butterfly arm action — entry

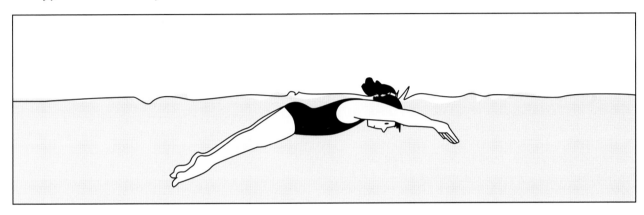

Butterfly arm action — catch

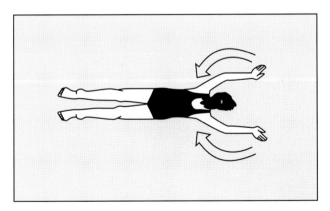

Butterfly arm action — insweep

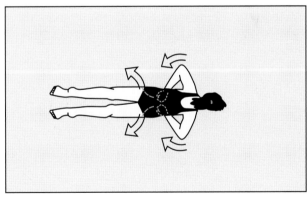

Butterfly arm action — upsweep

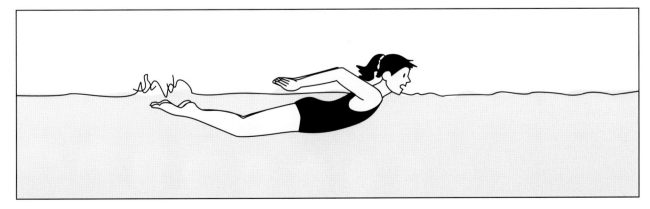

Butterfly arm action — recovery

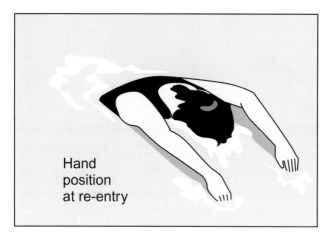

Butterfly arm action — hand position at re-entry

Breathing

The breathing action should be as natural as possible, with students avoiding excessively deep breathing or holding the breath for too long. During the butterfly stroke, students look to the front to inhale through the mouth, as the arms push underwater. The head should begin to be raised as the arms begin to sweep outwards during the catch. The face breaks the surface of the water during the push and upsweep of the arms and a breath is taken while the arms are fully supporting the student — prior to the recovery phase of the stroke. As the arms complete the recovery, the head slowly drops back into the water and exhalation occurs.

Coordination of the stroke

One arm stroke, two complete kick cycles and a breath constitute one stroke. Initially one kick per arm stroke is what is taught. It is considered important for students to have a pause between each arm stroke to allow the timing of the arms and legs to synchronise. The very slight glide or rest in the arm action allows the legs to complete the second downward kick.

Drills for students

ARM ACTION PRACTICES

With the use of a pull-buoy:
- one-arm practices
- right arm — one stroke
- left arm — one stroke
- students gradually increase the number of strokes from one to six with each arm.

With dolphin kick:
- one-arm practices as performed with a pull-buoy.

Combination arm drills:
- one right arm, one both arms and one left arm
- two right arm, two both arms and two left arm
- any other combination of arm practices may be included as performance improves.

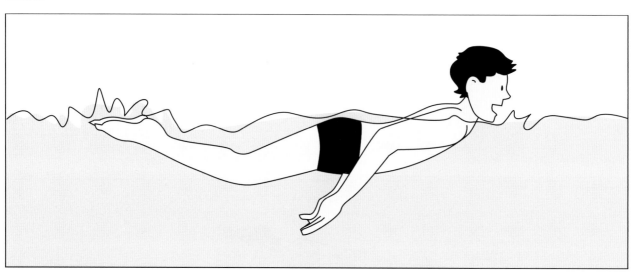

Butterfly breathing

Progressions

SUGGESTED STEPS

1. Dolphin kick underwater

Be cautious of head hitting the bottom of the pool.

a   On front, arms by sides.
b   Arms extended forward:
- undulating body
- head-leads movement
- legs kick together
- toes turn in
- lack of excessive knee bend.

2. Dolphin kick on surface

On the back:

a   arms by sides
b   arms extended forward
- emphasis on the up-beat (towards the surface).

On the front:

a   arms by sides
b   arms extended forwards
- emphasis on the down-beat (towards the bottom of the pool).

3. Arm action — without breathing

a   On land (leaning forwards).
b   In water (leaning forwards).
c   Swimming (short repetitions):
- arms at shoulder-width, thumbs down
- outward press
- inward pull under chest
- backward and outward push into recovery
- back of hand leading wide recovery.

4. Combining arm and leg action — without breathing

- Glide after first kick
- Push during second kick
- Short repetitions.

5. Combining breathing with arm and leg action

- Head lifting for breath during the push phase.
- Face looking forwards for breath.
- Face down for the hand entry.
- Shoulders remain low.

May be repeated, ideally breathing every second stroke.

Option

One-arm drills:
- breathing to the side initially
- dolphin kick
- butterfly arm recovery
- unused arm extended forwards.

May be repeated, breathing every second stroke.

Many combinations may be created using right arm, left arm, double arm, etc.

Option

Whole stroke with extra kick(s) (e.g. two kicks in a glide position before the arm action commences).

6. Whole stroke

- Glide after first kick.
- Push during second kick.

7. Refine the stroke

Continue refining the individual components of the stroke.

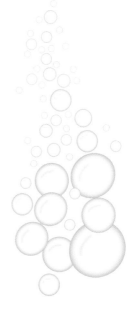

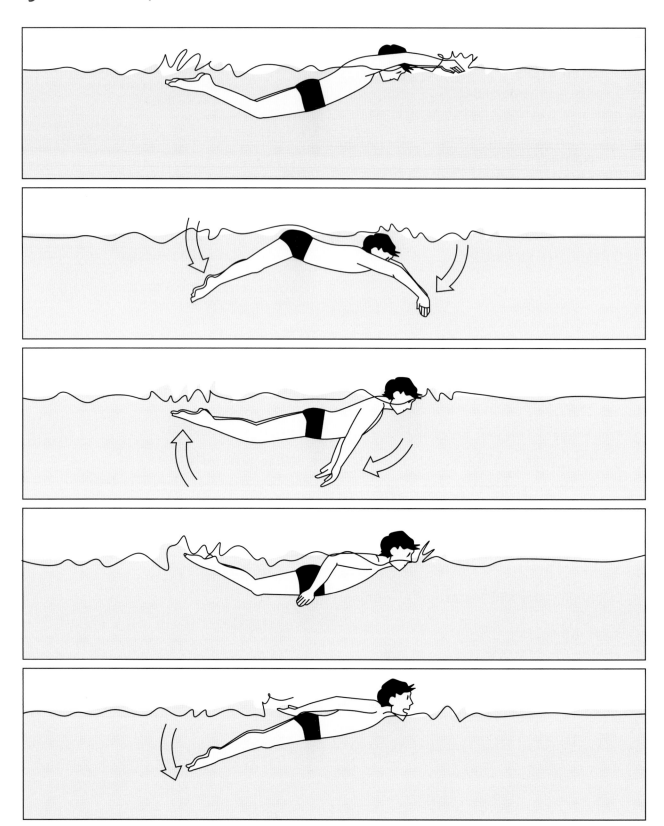

Butterfly sequence

Evaluating technique

The overall timing, or flow, of the stroke is more important than precision of the details. Remember that butterfly is an involved stroke. All its parts fit together and all are necessary.

Look for the features listed below.

BODY POSITION

Watch for a constantly undulating torso. Students should be attempting to poke their buttocks out of the water as their hands enter and glide downwards to a depth of about 20 cm.

ARM ACTION

- Emphasise variation in arm speed — slow pull, fast push and swing wide, with a slight pause in front for the catch.
- For the arm entry, see that the arms are loosely extended, with the elbows slightly flexed and pointed upwards. The hands are rotated thumb-side down to about a 30/45 degree angle on entry — 90 degree on recovery.
- Emphasise that the arm pull is started by flexing the wrists. Make sure that the arm pull does not start until the kick has pushed the buttocks to the surface and the shoulders are 5–6 cm below the surface.
- Make sure the hands are near the surface, out of the student's line of sight, as the pull begins. See that the pull begins gently, with the forearms descending and the elbows remaining high, just below the surface.
- The pull should not begin until there are 5–6 cm of water over the shoulders.
- Emphasise that the pull scribes a keyhole or hourglass shape. See that the push ends with the thumbs about even with the leg-line of the swimsuit. Also, at the end of the push, see that the arms rotate from the shoulders to turn the palms inwards.
- Emphasise that the arms are bent at a right angle, the elbows pointing outwards, during most of the pull.
- During the recovery phase of the arm action, see that the arms are not rigid and that the hands are relaxed. The elbows lift out first, followed by the hands.

LEG ACTION

- Watch for the knees bending, leading both the down-beat and the up-beat. The feet and ankles should break the surface of the water before each kick. For the down-beat the knees should be about 15 cm apart and the feet should be pigeon-toed.
- Emphasise a slight pause after each up-beat, with legs high and streamlined.
- Emphasise two kicks per cycle — a kick when the head goes under and a kick when the head comes out. Kick on catch and kick on push (upsweep of hands).
- Check that the hips are high, that the legs are working relatively high in the water and that the head and shoulders are going below with each entry.
- Look for symmetry in the arm and leg movements.

HEAD POSITION

- Watch for the smooth movements of the head, with the jaw thrust forward and low.
- For the head–hands timing, see that the head is lifted out before the hands and put back into the water before the hands re-enter the water in front. The head should start to rise when the hands are about a quarter of the way through the underwater stroke.

BREATHING

- Inhalation should be completed during the last half of the push phase and during the first half of the arm recovery. Students should breathe out through the mouth and nose into the water. Students should be encouraged to perform extended breathing on every second stroke, or more if comfortable.

Checklist for evaluating beginner butterfly

- ❑ Good streamlined body position.
- ❑ Undulating body position throughout the kicking action.
- ❑ Kick initiated from the hips, legs together with simultaneous movement.
- ❑ Kick extended through the legs and ankles.
- ❑ Simultaneous and continuous arm movement (keyhole pattern).
- ❑ Relaxed arm action on recovery.
- ❑ Breath is taken during the last part of the push phase prior to recovery of the arms.

Principles of movement in water for butterfly

RESISTANCE

Butterfly is like 'double-arm freestyle', but is slower than freestyle because its wider outsweep and deeper knee bend create greater frontal resistance. The symmetrical arm and leg movements can cause rapid fatigue because great strength is required from the upper body for the double-arm recovery.

Students need to practise dolphin-like movement — a natural undulating movement helps to produce natural speed. Various elementary drills to encourage good flexion from the hips and an efficient dolphin kick are necessary to gain effective propulsion.

Excessive flexion of the hips and head creates frontal resistance and is a common problem with students. The use of fins is encouraged to help students achieve the undulating movement required. The head acts as a control point of the body and any excessive head movement will cause resistance.

PROPULSION

Key considerations for efficient butterfly include the following:

1   The arms glide down to a depth of 20 cm as they begin the outsweep. The thumbs point downwards as the palms face outwards. Effective sculling during the outsweep and insweep provides the lift that is required to breathe properly and will assist in the undulating movement of the body. The outsweep is very important in setting up a strong insweep that enhances the speed of the arm pull.

2   The final sweep of the butterfly, referred to as the upsweep, produces the greatest power in the arm action. This phase also produces lift and blends in with the previous insweep phase. The head breaks the surface of the water during the upsweep and full inhalation occurs when the arms start to recover. The breath is taken when the body produces the greatest amount of lift, therefore not disrupting the natural flow of the butterfly stroke. This action prevents greater turbulence and frontal resistance.

3   The above-water arm recovery of butterfly should cleanly enter the water, with the hands entering at approximately 45 degrees to minimise turbulence. A slightly bent arm recovery is recommended to enable a clean entry in line with the shoulders. It is quite acceptable for swimmers to adopt a straight-arm recovery and it will work efficiently if the entry is clean and the shoulder joint speed is relatively fast.

4   The kick works in unison with the upper body, so the dolphin-like action of the body is coordinated efficiently. The down-beat provides the drive and occurs as the hands enter the water and again as the hands leave the water. There must be two kicks per stroke cycle so that the stroke maintains acceleration. Like freestyle and backstroke, the kick must originate from the hips to produce maximum force. The knees simply bend to assist in the body's undulating action. As the hands enter the water the buttocks come out of the water because the hips flex to assist in the dolphin-like action.

Legs and feet

The legs work in symmetry to produce efficient movement. The dolphin kick has been proven to be the most effective underwater kick because the paired leg action creates less turbulence. As in freestyle, the down-beat provides the drive, but the knee bend is slightly deeper to promote the undulating action and to provide greater stability as the arms exit and recover. Good hip-flexion is the key to an efficient kick and the legs should be allowed to move naturally from the undulating movement of the upper body.

Summary

Butterfly has evolved in recent years as coaches have attempted to break records by encouraging swimmers to travel underwater for a long distance. (Federation Internationale de Natation Amateur rules limit the distance to a maximum of 15 m.) Turbulence and eddies are created when the body is on the surface and more splash is produced. Swimming underwater minimises these resistances but only an extremely effective kick will produce good speed. After a freestyle tumble-turn, the dolphin kick is used instead of the flutter kick. As humans have studied the efficient movements of marine life, they have adopted the improved techniques to increase speed. Butterfly is a classic example: it aims to simulate the movement patterns of the dolphin.

SIDESTROKE

Clear vision in the direction of travel and uninterrupted breathing are features of this stroke. Each limb action follows a different movement pathway, but as the actions are similar to natural movements encountered in everyday life, sidestroke is not a difficult stroke to master.

Most students will start on a preferred side, but it is desirable that students should be able to perform sidestroke on both sides.

Body position

Body position in the glide is directly on the side with the lower arm extended beyond the head and the upper arm resting along the side of the body.

Leg action

Sidestroke leg action is called the scissor kick.

THE RECOVERY

From the glide position, the legs bend together to a position where they form a triangle shape with the hips at the apex.

The legs then separate, with the top leg (i.e. the leg nearest the surface of the water) moving forwards, the knee slightly flexed and the foot dorsi-flexed. The action is similar to taking a big forward step.

At the same time, the lower leg is extended backwards, knee slightly flexed and foot plantar-flexed (pointed), like a big backward step.

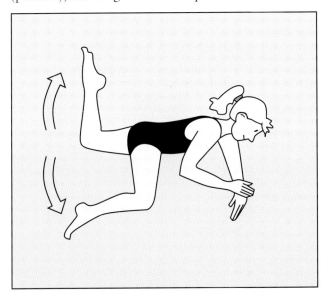

Sidestroke leg action — recovery

THE KICK

From this wide position the feet are swept together in an accelerating circular motion. The foot of the top leg initiates the movement by whipping into plantar-flexion as both legs straighten and sweep outwards and around before coming together in the glide position.

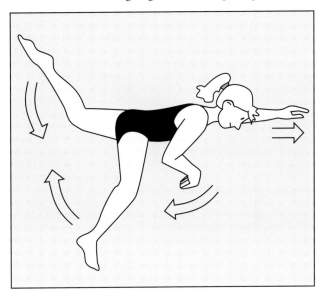

Sidestroke leg action — propulsion

THE GLIDE

The student holds the glide position and rests until the forward movement of the body slows, then the next stroke cycle is begun. The glide, or rest phase, is a most important part of this stroke in survival situations, allowing the body to rest and therefore increase endurance time. During competition, the glide is reduced to maximise time spent on active propulsion.

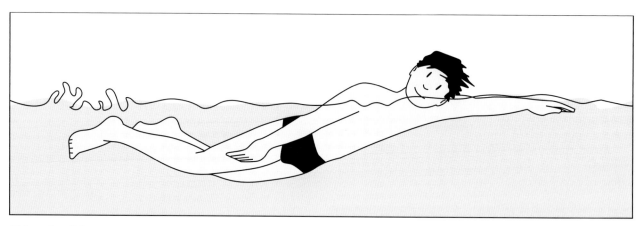

Sidestroke glide

Arm action

In sidestroke each arm follows a different movement pathway. The action begins from the glide position with the propulsive action of the lower arm and the recovery of the upper arm.

THE LOWER ARM

Propulsion

The wrist of the lower arm flexes as the hand catches the water; the elbow bends as the hand sweeps in a curved pathway slightly in front of the body-line to the shoulder.

Recovery

The lower arm recovers in a spear-like action, extending directly towards the direction of travel while maintaining maximum streamlining, palm down.

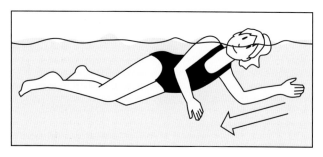

Propulsive phase of the lower arm, the legs are recovering

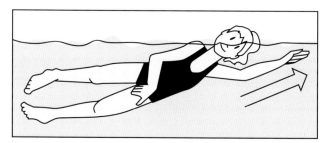

The lower arm recovers as the legs propel the body forward

THE UPPER ARM

Recovery

The elbow and wrist flex to allow the hand to move up beside the body to a position in front of the lower shoulder, where the wrist straightens and the hand extends. The arm and hand remain as close to the body as possible during recovery, to maximise streamlining.

Propulsion

From this bent-arm position the hand turns away from the body and pushes in a curved pathway to the thigh, ending in the glide position.

Timing

As the lower arm propels, the upper arm recovers, then continues the propulsive action while the lower arm recovers. This cycle is followed by the glide.

The upper arm works in conjunction with the legs, both recovering and propelling at the same time. The lower arm works in opposition to this, propelling as the arms and legs recover.

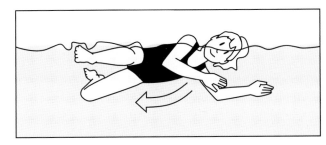

The upper arm provides propulsion to assist the kick, while the lower arm recovers

Breathing

Although the face may be held clear of the water, this position increases resistance, so students should master a simple and efficient breathing technique. In sidestroke, the head rests on the lower shoulder with the face underwater and exhalation takes place during the propulsive phase of the upper arm and legs. While gliding, the face is turned upwards, clear of the surface, and the breath taken. The head turns back to rest on the shoulder, the face is submerged, and the next stroke cycle commences.

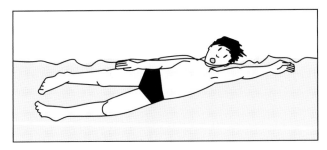

Sidestroke breathing

Coordination of the stroke

As students sometimes find it difficult to maintain a stable position on the side while floating, it may be helpful to use aids such as kickboards to assist stability when practising leg action.

THE LEG ACTION

After demonstration on land, in the water and perhaps on video, the leg action should be attempted. Keywords may help students with the sequence.

Bend

Legs remain together and bend to initiate the recovery action.
   Check that:
- legs are together
- legs form a triangle.

Open

Legs separate forwards and backwards in giant stride.
   Check that:
- position is wide
- knees are slightly flexed
- top leg is forwards
- top foot is dorsi-flexed
- lower foot is plantar-flexed
- movement is in horizontal plane.

Kick

Legs sweep outwards and around and finish together.
   Check that:
- top foot becomes plantar-flexed
- kick is circular and accelerating
- movement stops when feet meet.

Glide

Legs are straight and are held together.
   Check that:
- legs are straight
- toes are pointed
- body is directly on the side.

THE ARM ACTION

The arm action may be practised in the water while the beginner walks through the water, leaning slightly sideways towards the direction of travel with the lower shoulder in the water.
   Check that:
- arm actions are 'opposite' (i.e. one recovers as the other pulls)
- the propulsive action has a fluid changeover from the lower arm to the upper arm.

THE INVERTED SCISSOR KICK

This faulted kick is performed when the upper leg moves backwards in the recovery when the legs separate. Turning the student onto the other side may correct this fault initially, but as it is desirable that students perform sidestroke on both sides, it is important that time is spent in perfecting the correct action on both sides. Note: In some rescues the inverted scissor kick may be used to advantage to facilitate towing.
   Once sidestroke is mastered, practices should include:
- distance swimming on either side to increase endurance
- rescue activities — towing a number of partners of different body size and buoyancy, under a range of water and weather conditions, over increasing distances.

Progressions

It is recommended that the teaching of sidestroke is left until a symmetrical leg action in breaststroke has been well established. If it is not established, negative transfer of learning may occur, leading to a crooked scissor action during the breaststroke kick. However, sidestroke has great value in survival and rescue situations and should not be neglected.

SUGGESTED STEPS

1. Leg action lying on side (in very shallow water)

From a position with legs extended:
a. Bend:
  - legs bend together at hip and knee
  - bend at hips to 45 degrees.
b. Open:
  - upper leg moves forwards — toes back
  - lower leg moves back — toes pointed
  - wide position
  - movement in horizontal plane only.
c. Kick:
  - circular, accelerating action
  - toes of upper foot become pointed
  - upper and lower legs straighten
  - movement in horizontal plane only
  - movement stops when feet meet.
d. Glide:
  - pause for glide phase
  - legs straight and together
  - toes pointed.

2. Glide on the side

In a horizontal body position on side:
- ear in water
- lower arm extended forwards
- upper arm extended backwards
- legs together with toes pointed.

3. Leg action swimming on side

With board(s):
- lower arm extended forwards (with board)
- upper arm extended back (with board)
- ear in water
- horizontal body position on side
- significant glide phase.

Option

Add lower arm action to Step 3 above.

4. Arm action

Standing or leaning sideways in water:
- lower hand pulling towards shoulder while upper hand recovers towards shoulder
- lower arm recovering forwards while upper arm pushes towards the thigh.

5. Coordination of whole stroke

Standing:
- pulling with lower arm while upper arm and upper leg recover
- kicking and pushing with upper arm while lower arm recovers
- pause for the glide phase.

Swimming:
- horizontal body position on side
- ear in water
- arm action, leg action and timing as above.

6. Refine the stroke

Continue refining the individual components of the stroke.

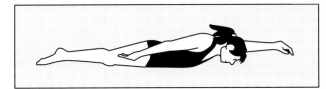

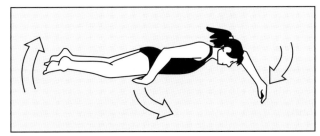

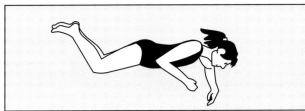

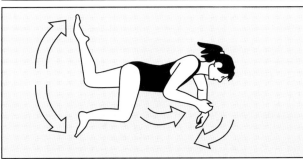

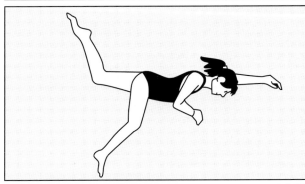

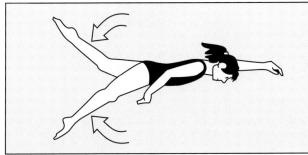

Sidestroke sequence

Evaluating technique

Look for the following features:
- the limb actions are smooth and coordinated
- the body is directly on the side
- the ear is resting on the lower shoulder
- the face is angled slightly upwards
- the arms work in opposite directions
- wide leg action
- circular, accelerating kick
- top leg forward — foot dorsi-flexed
- movement mainly in horizontal plane
- feet meet and remain together for glide
- the glide is held for one to two seconds
- legs and upper arm work together.

Principles of movement in water for sidestroke

RESISTANCE

Sidestroke is the only stroke in which the body is on its side. The body position is streamlined, on its side, with the lower arm extended beyond the head.

As one arm recovers and the legs adopt the scissor kick action, significant frontal resistance is created. The wide, sweeping action of the legs in the recovery phase creates a slow stroke, but the fast 'snapping' action of the legs in the propulsive phase produces good speed.

The arms work in unison, one arm always providing propulsion as the other arm recovers. Like survival backstroke, the recovering arm 'slides' through the water to minimise eddies and frontal resistance. The effective sculling actions of the arms and hands attempt to maximise forward movement but this can only happen when there is no patient in tow.

PROPULSION

Key considerations for efficient sidestroke include the following:

1. The elbows bend in the propulsive phases of both arms to generate maximum power, assisting the legs to increase speed. The face of each hand opens to effectively catch the water and propel the body forwards. When the hands open up to 'grip' the water, this results in positive drag. As the arms extend, the body travels past the point where the water was caught.

2. The powerful closure of the legs in the propulsive phase of the scissor kick is the source of optimal movement in the stroke. The top leg (i.e. the leg closest to the surface of the water) comes forward and the foot is dorsi-flexed. The back of the top

leg and the sole of the foot catch the water and propel the body forwards. The bottom leg flexes from the knee and the toe is angled away from the body. The toe is pointed (plantar-flexed), producing a strong hold on the water to maximise propulsion.

3   If the arm action and leg action fail to coordinate, the stroke will create turbulence because the struggle to synchronise the stroke will produce disturbed water. To improve coordination the arm action can be performed with just one arm working with the legs, and land drills of the action can be practised.

4   The glide phase is streamlined, with the bottom arm extended and the top arm positioned on the thigh. The head must rest on the water's surface, with the cheek and ear in the water. A raised head produces an inclined body position which will increase frontal resistance. It can also cause turbulence because the angle of the legs will produce an ineffective kick. The body must travel in the horizontal plane to prevent further resistance.

SURVIVAL BACKSTROKE

This stroke is an easy stroke to master and is usually taught in conjunction with breaststroke. As with any symmetrical movements, it is important to emphasise the symmetry, particularly the leg action. There is no vision in the direction of travel, so students should be encouraged to use landmarks as guidelines to direction.

Body position

Body position is on the back with the body straight and the arms by the sides in the glide position.

Leg action

The leg action is the inverted whip kick.

THE RECOVERY

From the extended position of the glide, the legs bend at the knees and drop to assume a vertical position with the feet dorsi-flexed and averted. The knees are slightly parted, but no wider than the swimmer's shoulders.

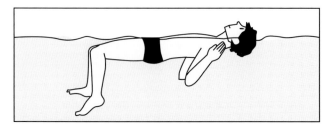

Survival backstroke leg sequence — recovery

THE KICK

The feet are swept in an accelerating circular motion, outwards, backwards and upwards, ending with the feet together, plantar-flexed, in the glide position. The movement is symmetrical and simultaneous.

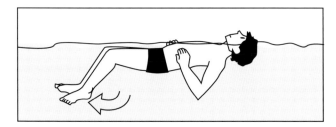

Survival backstroke leg sequence — kick

THE GLIDE

The swimmer maintains the streamlined glide position until the momentum of the body decreases.

Arm action

The arm action, like the leg action, is also symmetrical and simultaneous. The propulsive phases of both arms and legs occur at the same time.

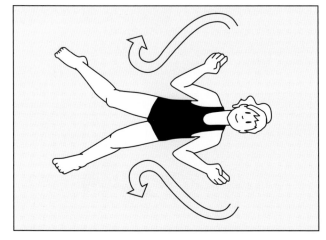

Survival backstroke — arm action for recovery

THE RECOVERY

From the extended arm position at the side of the body in the glide, the arms bend at the wrist and elbow to allow the hands to move to shoulder level while remaining very close to the body, 'thumbs along the rib cage'. It is important to keep the hands and arms close to the sides of the body to enhance streamlining. When the hands reach shoulder level, they extend beyond the shoulders, elbows bent, with hands facing away from the body and towards the feet.

From this position at the end of recovery, the arms follow a curved pathway until the hands and arms reach the glide position.

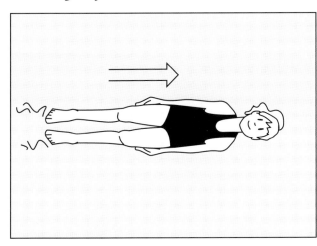

Arms and legs moving together to complete the glide for survival backstroke

Breathing

Breathing is natural — usually exhalation occurs with propulsion.

Coordination of the stroke

It is often useful to teach the inverted whip kick with the aid of a kickboard held to the chest to assist buoyancy and to enable the beginner to slow down and concentrate on the correct leg action.

Keywords may help the beginner with the sequence.

BEND

Legs bend at the knee and feet dorsi-flex.
Check that:
- the body is streamlined, on the surface, from the head through to the knees
- the knees are no more than shoulder-width apart
- the feet are turned out
- the body is symmetrical.

KICK

Legs move in a circular pathway.
Check that:
- the kick is circular
- the kick is accelerating
- the feet finish together, toes pointed, knees straight
- knees are under the surface
- the movement is symmetrical.

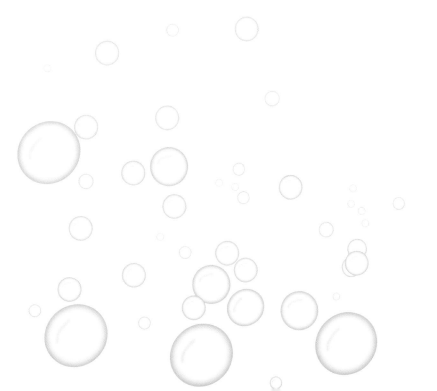

Progressions

The leg actions for survival backstroke and for breaststroke are largely identical. They differ only with regard to the degree of hip-flexion employed, survival backstroke using slightly less.

SUGGESTED STEPS

1. Foot exercises

Sitting, with legs extended:

- toes point down
- feet turn out ('hooked' position).

2. Backward glide and recovery

From a gliding position (shoulders under, head back):

- horizontal body position
- head submerged to the crown
- chin slightly tucked in
- recovery to a standing position.

Teach the recovery first.

3. Leg action on back (with board or sculling)

From a gliding position:

- glide, single kick, glide
- number of kicks gradually increasing
- toes turn out before kick
- shoulders, hips and knees horizontal
- limited hip-flexion
- glide between kicks.

4. Arm action

- arms recovering close to body
- palms pointing outwards (at shoulder level)
- hands pushing out and down to thighs.

Option

Basic arm action:

- shorter arm recovery
- simple push to the thigh.

5. Whole stroke

From a glide:

- arms start recovery just before legs
- arms and legs start push together
- significant glide phase.

6. Refine the stroke

Continue refining the individual components of the stroke.

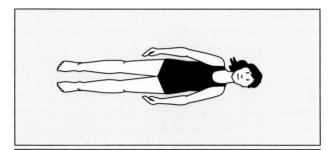
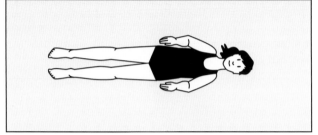
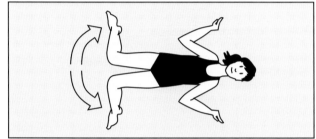
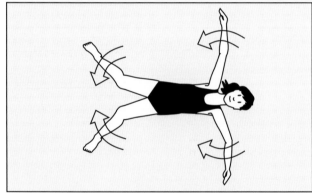
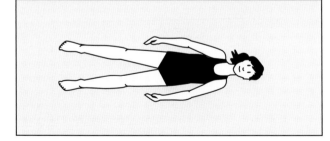

Survival backstroke sequence

Evaluating technique

Look for the following features:
- the propulsive actions of the arms and the legs are simultaneous
- the arm recovery begins slightly before that of the legs
- the body remains symmetrical throughout the whole stroke
- the glide is sustained
- the head position is in line with the body, with the face clear of the water
- the knees remain below the surface of the water
- the combined action of arms and legs provides strong propulsion.

Once survival backstroke has been mastered, students should practise the stroke over increasing distances, while wearing clothes, and while towing people of different size and buoyancy. Multiple rescues should also be practised. These activities should be undertaken under a variety of natural aquatic conditions.

Principles of movement in water for survival strokes

RESISTANCE

The survival strokes encounter greater resistance than the competitive strokes because of underwater recovery actions. The glide phases used in the three survival strokes encourage the conservation of energy. However, efficient arm and leg actions can speed up rescues and assist with the stabilisation of the victim.

Like breaststroke, survival backstroke experiences considerable frontal resistance due to the kicking action. The survival backstroke kick is the reverse copy of the breaststroke kick. The body position is horizontal, with the back on the water's surface, and the swimmer is encouraged to keep as close to the water's surface as possible. The sculling actions of the arms also create significant frontal resistance and turbulence. The sweeping action of the hands during arm recovery causes deceleration.

PROPULSION

Key considerations for efficient survival backstroke are:
1. The arm recovery will create frontal resistance, but if the hands 'slide' through the water towards the shoulders, it will minimise resistance. The arm can be compared to an oar, the blade of which is the hand. Opening the face of the hand produces maximum speed in the propulsive phase of the arm action, and the hand changes its angle during the recovery phase — exactly the same action as an oar.
2. The hands finish next to the thighs at the end of the push, to maximise distance per stroke and to encourage streamlining in the glide phase. The elbows bend during the propulsive phase to maximise the power generated from the upper body. The paired arm action in the propulsive phase can be compared to the backstroke action, but the hands do not extend far beyond the shoulders in survival backstroke.
3. The leg action starts with a bend at the knee joint to drop the lower legs (leg recovery) to set up the propulsive phase. It is common for students to flex their hips so the knees break the water. This action increases frontal resistance and causes eddy turbulence to form around the legs, close to the water's surface. If this action occurs, the body position will incline and result in an inefficient movement.
4. When the lower legs are dropped, ready for the propulsive phase, the ankles dorsi-flex and are positioned to 'grab' the water, and the legs extend and follow a semicircular path to maximise propulsion. It is important to realise that the leg rotation comes from the hip and not the knee. The knees start the propulsive action 30 cm apart, which assists the lower legs to rotate efficiently.
5. The legs finish in an extended position for a streamlined glide phase. The toes are pointed (plantar-flexed) to minimise frontal resistance. The stroke cycle continues.

Correctional strategies

FAULT	CORRECTION
Body position	
Head too high — freestyle, breaststroke, butterfly, backstroke	• Practise streamlining skills • Use kickboard • Ensure that water is across forehead/hairline • Check hip position and knee bend • Work on efficiency of stroke as often the fault is due to a lift of the head for breathing purposes • Ask student to slightly look forwards underwater (head down further in freestyle and breaststroke, water across forehead) • Ask student to look up at approximately 45 degrees in backstroke, head level, eyes looking back above feet
Head too deep — freestyle, breaststroke, butterfly, backstroke	• Practise streamlining skills • Use kickboard • Ensure that water is across forehead/hairline • Check hip position and knee bend — often hips are bent forwards with body in sitting position in freestyle or butterfly • Ask student to look forward slightly, underwater, in freestyle and breaststroke • Ask student to look up at approximately 45 degrees in backstroke
Body not streamlined — all strokes	• Practise streamlining skills • Check head position • Check hip position and legs • Ensure kicks are small movements without excessive hip bend, even in breaststroke
Legs too low in water — freestyle	• Practise kicking drills with no kickboard • Small flutter kicks • Avoid excessive knee bend • Waterline must remain on forehead, eyes look forwards • The position of the eyes have more impact than extreme movements of the head
No body roll — freestyle, backstroke	• Practise kicking and rolling from side to side during streamlining drills and also with kickboard • Exaggerate shoulder lifting and keeping head stable during kicking drills with and without kickboard
Leg action—FREESTYLE	
Excessive knee bend	• Practise kicking drill on land to minimise leg bend or hip-flexion • Small fast flutter kicks • Kick seated on wall, kick holding wall
Toes not pointed	• Practise kicking drill on land to minimise leg bend, and point toes • Ask student to practise this at home while watching TV or on a bed • Small fast flutter kicks — pointing toes • Kick seated on wall, kick holding wall

FAULT	CORRECTION
Leg action—BACKSTROKE	
Excessive knee bend (bicycle)	• In water kicking on back with kickboard over knees not touching board • Land drill with hips lifted slightly on kickboard • Flicking feet not pedalling
Toes not pointed	• Practise kicking drill on land on towel to minimise leg bend, and pointing toes • Ask student to practise this at home while watching TV or on a bed • Small fast flutter kicks — pointing toes
Leg action—BREASTSTROKE	
Feet not turned out during propulsive phase	• Land drill with knees slightly apart and feet together during out-push (propulsive phase) — penguin walk • Pushing off side wall with the ball of the foot
No glide at end of kick	• Pause kick phase at end of each kick • Ask student to touch big toes together and hold them together for a count of one
Knees bending under body	• Practise kick on back with kickboard held on hips • Land practice lying on towel • Minimum hip-flexion
Screw kick	• Work along one wall pushing off with ball of foot and return along the wall • Work right then left leg this way • Seated on wall, practising • Physical manipulation (with care), dry land practice
Leg action—SIDESTROKE	
Breaststroke kick	• Don't introduce sidestroke too early
Dolphin kick/freestyle kick	• Land drill
Leg action—SURVIVAL BACKSTROKE	
Same as breaststroke	• Use same drills as breaststroke; these complement each other • Correction for one fixes problems with others
Knees up to chest	• Practise on front, on towel • Board over knees, emphasising heels to bottom • Over edge of pool, on back
Leg action—BUTTERFLY	
Flutter kick	• Underwater off a wall while streamlining • Short sharp kicks up and down
Too much knee bend	• Practise on land with kickboard under hips • Standing in water, just out from wall, moving hips backwards and forwards
Not symmetrical	• Do not practise at same time as doing freestyle drills

FAULT	CORRECTION
Arm action—FREESTYLE	
Enter little finger first	• Practise using a kickboard, placing hand on lower edge of the board
Entering across the midline of the body	• Practise using a kickboard, placing hand on lower edge of the board • Slow motion swimming (controlling body roll) • Fingertip drag
Entering too wide	• Practise using a kickboard, placing hand on lower edge of the board
Fingers apart — wide (beginners)	• This is often only due to excessive tension and will reduce as efficiency improves
Short arm pull	• Touch thigh before recovery • Push back at end of stroke
Short arm entry	• Remind learner to lift elbow out and rotate arm forwards • One-arm drill using a kickboard out the front and just touching it lightly with fingers
Arm action—BACKSTROKE	
Little finger exit first	• Practise back-of-hand exit, asking the student to drop the hand and relax the wrist
Hand enter too wide or too far across the midline	• Stress reaching above shoulder • Single-arm drill holding small kickboard above the head • Emphasise brushing ear with arm
Bent-arm recovery	• Reach high and touch thigh on push before starting recovery
Arm action—BREASTSTROKE	
Pulling back past shoulder line	• Promote fast stroke action with no pause, apart from in streamline position • Breaststroke arms with noodle under arms • Hands recover in front of chest • Use comparison to 'scraping out a large bowl'
Rest phase at end of pull phase	• Promote fast stroke action with no pause, apart from in streamline position • Breathe earlier (head up after arms out, head down with arms forward)
No glide	• Counting often works or ask student to hold streamline after kick phase • Kick — GLIDE — Pull — Breathe — then Kick again
Arm action—BUTTERFLY	
Arms not symmetrical	• Practise with NO breathing
Entering too wide	• Drop head to allow for arms to enter above head
Short exit	• Brush past hips, reminding student to touch hips with the thumb
Short entry	• Encourage straighter arm recovery
Arm action—SIDESTROKE	
Symmetrical arms Breaststroke arms	• Avoid practising at same time as learning breaststroke skills

FAULT	CORRECTION

Arm action—SURVIVAL BACKSTROKE

Entering propulsive phase too high above the head	• Soldier, monkey, aeroplane, SNAP

Breathing—FREESTYLE

Holding breath	• Work on bubbling practice • Static practice at side of pool • 'Humming' • Breathing patterns 1–2–breathe etc.
Looking forwards to breathe	• Chin touch shoulder or brushing shoulder
Excessive roll	• Check position of arm underwater; it is often pulling across the centre-line • Stroke drill using kickboard works for most students • Look at lane rope or pool gutter

Breathing—BACKSTROKE

Holding breath	• Blow sharp and fast • Breathe in on left and out on right — creates a rhythm

Breathing—BREASTSTROKE

Breathing too late in stroke	• Lift head as arms pull apart • Use an aid to assist with flotation • Start breathing at start of pull
Holding breath	• Long blow at end of arm pull/inward sweep • Reinforce a pattern in each cycle • Kick–glide–pull–breathe
Short exit	• Brush past hips, reminding student to touch hips with the thumb
Short entry	• Encourage straighter arm recovery

Breathing—BUTTERFLY

Breathing too late	• Lift head to breathe during propulsive phase of arm stroke • Breathing is earlier than most think • Need to commence breathing cycle at commencement of underwater pull phase
Breathing too early	• Work on rhythm • Commence breathing cycle at commencement of underwater pull phase

Breathing—SURVIVAL BACKSTROKE

Holding breath	• Reinforce a pattern in each cycle

Breathing—SIDESTROKE

Holding breath	• Reinforce a pattern in each cycle

FAULT	CORRECTION
Timing — FREESTYLE	
Stopping on arm exit at thigh	• Brush thigh as hand passes
Excessive catch-up	• Often due to excessive shoulder/head roll • Often caused by excessive use of incorrect drills • Promote continuous stroke, no pause or delay • Reverse catch-up • Make arms pause at opposite point
Timing — BACKSTROKE	
Stopping hands at side	• Brush thigh as hand passes • 4 left, 4 right, 4 normal, alternating — count as hand enters water, on 4 switch arms
One arm not opposite to other	• Reaching for catch helps keep cycle • Breathing in on left-arm movement and out on right-arm movement helps
Timing — BREASTSTROKE	
Pull starts before kick has finished	• Promote phases • Have student practise kick–glide–pull–breathe–kick
Arms and leg start at the same time	• Promote phases • Have student practise kick–glide–pull–breathe–kick
Timing — BUTTERFLY	
Not two kicks to one arm stroke	• This skill is advanced and will only come with practice leading to efficiency • First kick during start of pull and start second kick during recovery — teach timing out of water • One-arm butterfly (advanced students only) • Dry land practice — vertical
If not kicking on entry and before exit	• This needs to be practised without breathing • Teach timing out of water • Encourage big kicks — good undulations • Dry land practice
Timing — SIDESTROKE	
Pull and recovery of both arms not at the same time	• Practise pulling along a rope, one hand at a time, or simulate this • Pick the apple, put it in the other hand, put it in the basket • Encourage glide, make sure student starts stroke with arms fully extended • Dry land practice
Arms and legs not in time	• Dry land practice, and also promote a glide at end of kick to stop confusion
Timing — SURVIVAL BACKSTROKE	
Propulsive phase of both arms and legs not occurring at same time	• Again this is just practice and a glide phase needs to be reinforced

REVIEW QUESTIONS

1   Name the different types of swimming strokes and provide an example for when each might be used.

2   List and describe the following components of each stroke:

- body position
- leg action
- arm action
- breathing.

3   For each stroke, list and describe drills that can be used to help the student's technique.

4   What are the key points you should look for when evaluating the technique of each stroke?

5   What are some correctional strategies a teacher can use if their student's:

- head is too high or low in the water?
- body is not streamlined?
- legs are too low in the water?

Plan, deliver and
review a lesson

CHAPTER 10

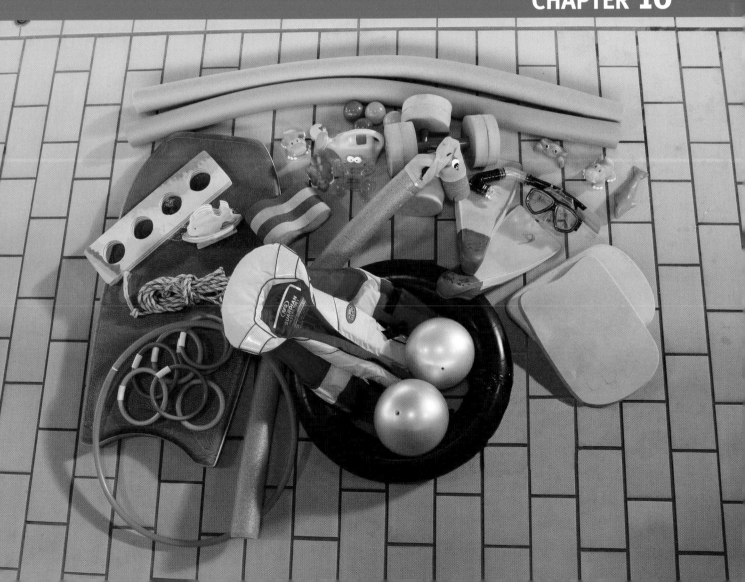

PLANNING A LESSON

The lesson plan is a major responsibility for the teacher. Students will soon sense hesitancy on the part of the teacher or will become bored with a lesson that has been inadequately prepared, and their attention will be lost. All segments of the lesson must be planned thoroughly in order to ensure safety, enjoyment and an efficient program.

Indeed, it may be said that *failing to prepare is preparing to fail.*

The lesson plan acts as a guide, giving the starting points and the steps needed to reach the goals that have been set. When developing a lesson plan it must be remembered that each student in the group is an individual, with different needs, abilities and possibly fears. Planning frequently involves a great deal of imagination as well as trial and error. Sometimes the lesson looks great in theory, but in practice may require some refinement or adjustment.

In addition, not only must the lesson be planned thoroughly, but alternatives must be prepared for varying conditions, such as inclement weather when teaching outdoors, disruptive students, lack of equipment, or a class that learns rapidly.

An overall structure that could be a basis for most lessons might include, first, a revision of the most recently learnt skills, then a (short) period teaching appropriate skill progressions and, finally, an enjoyable game involving all students practicing their new skills.

A more detailed breakdown of a typical lesson might contain:
- introduction
- revision (or assessment if first lesson)
- main skill set
- new skill set
- games
- conclusion.

Structure of a lesson

INTRODUCTION

Warm up activity = vigorous, fun, establishes theme.

REVISION/ASSESSMENT

Initial class is assessed; revise activities previously learnt; emphasise theme.

MAIN SKILL SET/NEW SKILL SET

- Extend known activities or introduce new activities.
- Introduction to variety of ways of performing activities; for example, at various depths; with a variety of equipment; with a partner.

GAMES

Select games relating to theme and new activities. Maximise fun element and participation.

CONCLUSION

Cool-down activity, reinforce lesson theme.

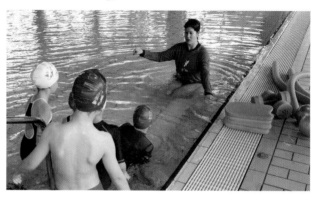

Plan your lesson

Setting objectives

The word 'objectives' is enough to strike fear in the heart of many teachers. In reality, objectives are simply steps through which to achieve an overall goal. Objectives must be:
- specific
- measurable
- achievable
- realistic
- time related.

They should be set for each class and for each individual in it. For example, after completing a beginners' program the students should be able to:
- wade confidently across the pool
- sit on the bottom
- blow bubbles while totally submerged
- have knowledge of and practise basic aquatic safety rules.

Subsequently, the more advanced student should be able to demonstrate:
- an understanding of water safety practices
- an understanding of buoyancy principles
- two methods of propulsion.

PROGRESSIVE STEPS

Once a set of objectives has been established, the next stage is to devise the steps required to achieve them. Using the previous example and establishing it for a set of lessons, the program plan may be as follows.

Step 1 Water entry via the steps and from sitting on the side; basic water safety.

Step 2 Practising known land skills in water: standing, walking, running, jumping, hopping.

Step 3 Steps towards confidence when immersing body and face.

Step 4 Buoyancy on front, back and sides.

Step 5 Body rotations: back to front to side to back.

Step 6 Push and glide with rotations and body steering.

Step 7 Mobility in leg and arm practices with and without an aid.

Step 8 Combinations of leg and arm practices.

This plan will establish a natural progression in the program, leading from the simple to the more difficult. Progress is made only as each objective is achieved, with some flexibility to promote variety.

The skills component

When developing the skills component a number of factors have to be considered, such as:

- the number in the group
- ability levels
- age and physical capabilities, including possible disabilities
- available equipment
- prevailing weather conditions
- size of the working area
- water conditions and temperature.

Medical considerations

Teachers of swimming and water safety must know the general medical condition of their students and also specific medical conditions if the latter are likely to cause risk to life or to create learning and teaching difficulties. In particular, students who suffer from any condition that may lead to loss of consciousness should (a) have medical clearance and (b) receive extra supervision.

The teacher should be familiar with common medical conditions prior to embarking on a program. Refer to Appendix 4.

LESSON SAFETY CHECKLIST

Use the following checklists as a guide to ensure you don't miss anything vital when planning your lessons.

FIRST LESSON

- ☐ Communicate with parents (proposed activities, dismissal time and place etc.).
- ☐ Check venue for hazards or potential dangers.
- ☐ Check all equipment/aids to ensure they are in good and safe condition.
- ☐ Check emergency/rescue equipment and first-aid facilities.
- ☐ Check enrolment (correct level/stage).
  - ☐ Create accurate class role.
  - ☐ Explain rules and emergency procedures.
  - ☐ Create a buddy system.
  - ☐ Point out important aspects of the venue (deep/dangerous/slippery etc.).
  - ☐ Assess ability in safety (and shallow water) to ensure in correct class.
  - ☐ Teach students the distress signal as soon as possible.
  - ☐ Pool rules.
  - ☐ Role of lifeguard (if applicable).
  - ☐ Parent/carer/school requirements (e.g. must stay poolside).

EVERY LESSON

- ☐ Have a rescue aid handy.
- ☐ Keep your class in view at all times.
- ☐ Organise equipment prior to the lesson.
- ☐ Check class list and record attendance.
- ☐ Check for medical and other considerations that may impact on a student's ability to participate.
- ☐ Check each student's attire (hair tied back, jewellery removed etc.).
- ☐ Ensure students have sun protection if outside (Note: Sunscreen must be applied by parent/carer, *not* AUSTSWIM teacher).
- ☐ Revise rules and emergency procedures.
- ☐ Revise whistle signals.
- ☐ Define boundaries.
- ☐ Check water quality and teaching equipment.
- ☐ Ensure privacy of class information.

DURING THE LESSON

- ☐ Check the number of students frequently.
- ☐ Control water entries and exits carefully.
- ☐ Create sufficient space for the individual.
- ☐ Avoid backward skills towards the pool edge (teach students about backstroke flags and their purpose).

(*lesson safety checklist* cont'd)

❑ Avoid backward skills in two directions.

❑ Conduct activities from deep to shallow rather than shallow to deep.

❑ Avoid activities that take your students through another class.

❑ Avoid formations that spread your class out around the venue.

❑ Avoid potentially dangerous areas (e.g. unsupervised diving boards).

❑ Arrange extra supervision if required (e.g. introduction to deep water).

❑ Use organised games for fun and use skill use/ extension rather than a 'free swim'.

❑ Do not dismiss your class prior to the end of the lesson.

❑ Ensure the students are handed over to their parent/teacher/guardian at the end of the lesson.

❑ If in doubt about an activity or situation, avoid it and seek advice.

DELIVERING A LESSON

Initial assessment

Assessment enables teachers to not only gain an understanding of each person's ability, but also to place students in classes according to ability. Similar ability groups are preferable so that lesson plans do not need to cover too wide a range of activities and skills, but are tailored to the needs of each group.

Flexibility

As already indicated, a well-prepared lesson should allow for flexibility. For instance, if students look bored, the teacher should change the activity or present it in an alternative way to provide encouragement and motivation. If they are showing interest it can be extended, gradually progressing to a related skill. An opportunity should not be missed just because the lesson plan has not included it.

Alternatively, if students are finding the skills too difficult, the teacher should revisit previously learnt skills then introduce the new skill (potentially in a different way).

For programs in outdoor or natural water environments, a resource kit for use in adverse weather conditions can be developed. It may include:

- videos showing stroke techniques and water safety or lifesaving skills (if facilities available)
- swimming and water safety topics for discussion
- a listing of dry-rescue techniques using a variety of aids

- fun activities associated with being near water
- basic life-support activities.

Catering for varying abilities

Although not preferable, there may be times when there will be students of different abilities in the one class. These differences may be in the form of swimming skills, intellectual capabilities or physical capabilities. The teacher is now required to set multiple lesson plans within the one class. This can be achieved by setting the same basic content and then extending or modifying the skill or distance of the skill for each student. A mixed-ability class can be advantageous to those students who are less capable as it gives them a standard to strive towards. This should be used to the teacher's advantage by using the more capable student as a demonstrator, or pairing those of different abilities together for some activities. The teacher also needs to be conscious of extending the more capable student so they don't stagnate. This can be done by working on the higher spectrum of skill performance.

The following progressions of streamlining are examples of how the same activity can be taught to different ability levels:

- push and glide with teacher assisting student by holding onto hands and guiding through the pool
- push and glide with arms extended using kickboard out in front for support
- push and glide with arms extended and hands locked together in streamlined body position
- push and glide with arms extended and hands locked together using flutter kick for 10 kicks.

The teacher needs to be vigilant in their supervision of this type of varied group as the less capable student may be tempted to perform skills above their ability level.

Being in or out of the water

This represents a common concern of many AUSTSWIM teachers and is a matter governed by one question: How many students can the teacher see at any given moment? Obviously, the answer has to be 'all of them'. If the teacher, when in water, can safely observe the entire class at all times, then this is considered permissible. However, to be in the water at the same level as the students, so that only a few of them can be seen, is considered an unsafe practice. The ability level of the student also needs to be taken into consideration as beginner-level students will need to have the teacher in the water with them.

Beginner to intermediate students benefit more and often respond better by having interaction with the teacher in the water. As long as supervision is maintained, students benefit from teacher demonstrations, communication on the same level, and a greater sense of safety and comfort.

TEACHING TIPS
- It is recommended when instructing in or out of the water that the teacher ensures that the students can be safely observed at all times.
- The teacher must be prepared to enter the water in the event of an emergency and therefore must be appropriately attired.

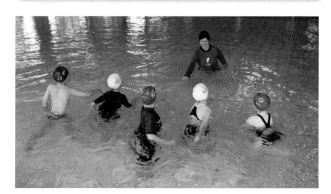

Conducting a lesson

Getting to know the students

Teachers should introduce themselves and ask the students their names. Trying to remember all those names on the first day is a feat in itself; however, it is a way of showing the students that they are important, and it is the first step in the development of a good relationship.

Also, the first day of a program is usually for assessment and possible regrouping, so it helps to know students' names rather than having to note that 'the little girl in the pink swimsuit needs to be in another group'. Once the group has settled down, it is appropriate to establish the rules regarding general behaviour and safety. All students must understand what is required of them, and teachers must remember the necessity to be consistent in their demands.

A 'challenge' for the teacher (which can also be an ice-breaker) is a game in which each student gives his or her name and then the teacher must try to recollect them all correctly. Each time a student is named, they must perform a skill (for example, jump high in the water, blow surface bubbles or submerge completely, according to ability).

Assessment

Assessment is an integral and ongoing part of any program and should be:
- informal
- continual.

It is important that teaching is directed to the needs of the students rather than to the requirements of any award scheme or certificate, which should be integrated into the program rather than allowed to direct it. Continual and informal assessment allows time to teach new skills and also to determine whether the students are learning the skills thoroughly and developing at their own rate.

After a student can perform a skill consistently and competently, the teacher may deem the skill as 'learnt'. With this method, each student progresses at his or her own pace and is not placed under too much pressure to advance.

Ultimately, it comes back to teachers knowing their students and deciding what is best for them to develop successfully.

Whenever possible, students should be assessed in groups rather than individually.

REVIEWING A LESSON

Continuous evaluation is essential for any successful program. Teachers must evaluate:

1 the lessons
2 each student
3 the program
4 their teaching performance.

Evaluating these four areas helps to identify problems in the program, enabling teachers to instigate a new approach or to make any changes if necessary. Teachers who strive for success will make evaluation an integral part of their planning.

LESSON EVALUATION

Some factors to be considered are:

- Was the group assessed correctly?
- Were the activities suitable for the ability and developmental needs of the class?
- Did each student benefit from the activities?
- Did the time allow for what had been planned?
- Were the students active throughout the lesson?
- Did the lesson run smoothly?
- Was the equipment readily available and easily accessible?
- Were the objectives achieved?

Student evaluation

This needs to be progressive, because students might not be able to proceed to a new skill until the previous one has been learnt. Evaluations should not be formal and are often better done without the student's knowledge, both to prevent the extra pressure created by formal testing and to minimise the time taken. Too much testing detracts from maximum learning and practice time; the class should be active for as much of the lesson time as possible.

Some factors to be considered are:

- Did the students appear interested in what they were doing?
- Did they understand everything that was asked of them?
- Is each one progressing successfully?
- Are they all enjoying what they are doing and having fun?
- Are they ready to progress to the next skill?

Program evaluation

As each program is completed, it should be evaluated in terms of the objectives set. For example, if the majority of the students did not reach the objectives, were those objectives unrealistic with respect to the students' physical and mental capabilities? If, on the other hand, all were successful, were the objectives too easily reached? Did they offer each student a satisfactory individual challenge?

This evaluation enables a teacher to identify the weaker areas of the program, allowing an opportunity to refine or eradicate these areas in future programs.

Evaluating teaching performance

Last, but by no means least, the teaching performance should be evaluated. A good teacher sets the atmosphere for a class: relaxing and enjoyable, as well as challenging and meaningful. One should be prepared to evaluate one's knowledge and performance, and should continually strive to keep abreast of modern developments.

The way a lesson is presented should also be evaluated; for example, did the teacher:

- talk too long?
- use words that students did not understand?
- become impatient?
- treat teaching with such seriousness that there were few smiles from the students?

If there is any question about the standard of teaching performance, it would be wise to reconsider the guidelines given in Chapter 4, 'Being an effective teacher'.

Some teachers of swimming and water safety challenge themselves constantly; others are prepared to teach in the same, unvaried way year after year. Some have had five years of teaching experience, but others have one year repeated five times!

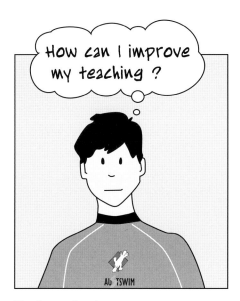

Teacher evaluation

STUDENT–TEACHER RATIOS

In planning a safe and successful swimming and water safety program it is important to group students, where possible, according to similar ability. It is also essential to follow established guidelines regarding student–teacher ratios and appropriate water depths. A copy of the AUSTSWIM recommended student–teacher ratios can be obtained from AUSTSWIM at www.austswim.com.au.

> **TEACHING TIPS**
> – The younger the child and the deeper the water, the greater will be the supervision required.
> – The ratios for open-water teaching venues were formulated after considering the following risk factors: angle of depth increase, minimum wave action, and current flow.

TEACHING EQUIPMENT

A teaching aid is anything that a teacher brings to a class that assists students with the learning of a skill. Aids can be extremely useful and enable students to practise a desired skill with less fatigue. Teachers should be prepared to patiently lead students through a range of progressive activities supplemented with incidental use of a variety of equipment. This will gradually increase students' understanding and recognition that the water will support them, with or without artificial support.

With timid or poorly coordinated students, flotation aids may help to obtain sufficient control and balance to maintain a buoyant position. The use of different flotation aids is important, but dependence on them should be reduced systematically and eliminated as soon as possible.

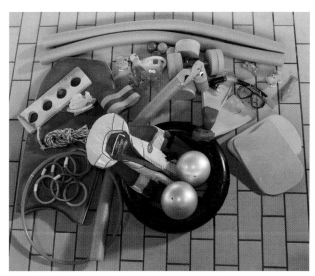

Teaching equipment

Advantages of teaching equipment

The use of teaching equipment should either make learning more enjoyable or provide students with a temporary physical boost that helps them to concentrate on and achieve a particular skill level.

Examples of each purpose are easy to find. A toy can be used to encourage a hesitant child to immerse the face in an attempt to recover the toy, and may also help in developing an understanding of buoyancy. Teaching aids, when used correctly, enable the student to maintain correct body position and breathe comfortably while a specific kick is learnt.

Disadvantages of teaching equipment

Overuse of teaching equipment occurs when a student is allowed to develop a dependency upon an aid, which either creates an impression that the skill in question cannot be performed without it or perhaps causes a fault in technique to develop. This sometimes occurs if a beginner always uses an aid to assist buoyancy and skills are never practised without it; the student believes that the aid is solely responsible for buoyancy.

Teachers and students should be made aware of the possible dangers of some teaching equipment. When using buoyancy aids such as flotation mats and large plastic toys it is possible for non-swimmers to be carried out of their depth by either wind or water action, thereby creating an extremely hazardous situation.

Teaching equipment in poor condition can be dangerous — for example, plastic kickboards that leak or have sharp edges, or bubbles with faulty clasps. Aids are an assistance, a means to an end; they are not ends in themselves. Used wisely, they will enhance the learning process, but used unwisely their effect is negative. Having given a student an aid, it is incumbent upon the teacher to devise appropriate strategies to withdraw it gradually, so that the student's confidence is not lost in the process.

Examples of types of equipment

INSTRUCTIONAL/ACTIVITY EQUIPMENT

- Kickboards
- Balls
- Plastic hoops
- Ice-cream containers (with drilled shower holes)
- Small buckets
- Dive rings
- Water flotation mats
- Flotation toys
- Water puppets
- Saturn water toys
- Water logs/noodles
- Small colourful toys
- Broom handles
- Platforms (to alter the depth of the water)

Please note for hygiene purposes avoid toys that retain water. Most importantly, students need teachers with imagination and enthusiasm.

SKILL DEVELOPMENT EQUIPMENT

- Fins/flippers
- Pull-buoys
- Hand and finger paddles
- Leg bands
- Drag suits

WATER SAFETY/RESCUE EQUIPMENT

- Kickboards
- Boogie boards
- Balls
- Inner tubes
- Water logs/noodles
- Pull-buoys
- Rescue poles
- Buckets
- Eskies (cool-storage container)
- Plastic containers
- Throw rope
- Goggles (personal)
- Plastic weighted hoops
- Plastic dive discs
- Dive rings
- Rubber bricks
- Flexible dive sticks

DRY ACTIVITIES EQUIPMENT

- Videos
- Posters
- Manikins

CONDUCTING A SAFE AQUATIC PROGRAM IN AN OPEN WATER ENVIRONMENT

Qualifications

Teachers working in natural water environments have to be particularly well prepared for emergencies. Communication and immediate access to assistance must be carefully and thoroughly considered.

AUSTSWIM teachers must maintain the currency of their AUSTSWIM, rescue and resuscitation qualifications. Teachers instructing in open water are required to hold the relevant rescue qualification for the environment in which they are teaching. The relevant award may be obtained from either the Royal Life Saving Society Australia (www.royallifesaving.com.au) or Surf Life Saving Australia (www.slsa.asn.au).

Lifesaving and resuscitation

Lifesaving, including rescue and resuscitation skills, are often neglected. It is the responsibility of teachers to hold current CPR qualifications.

Lesson area

The lesson area should be checked for depth, holes, snags, currents, slippery rocks or tiles, or any other likely hazard. In pools or other limited spaces, beginners should be set an area within which to attend lessons. A handy aid for defining areas in open water is a collection of plastic fruit juice containers tied to a weight, or tied to a floating rope and anchored at corner points. The containers can be positioned to define the teaching area limits for the class. In natural venues, floats of distinctive colours can be used to denote potential hazards that cannot be eliminated.

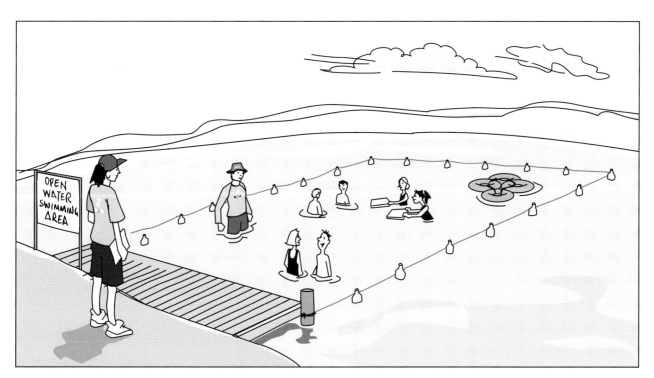

The lesson area

Secure rest stations

Secure rest stations, which may also be used in emergency situations, must be placed in selected areas. Tyre tubes firmly lashed together and anchored to the bottom will suffice if permanent pontoons are not available.

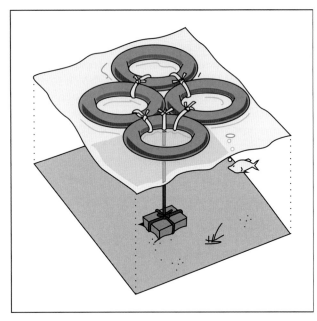

Secure rest stations

A manoeuvrable and quick rescue craft

A manoeuvrable and quick rescue craft is essential at natural water venues, even if the water is shallow. A stable craft, such as a surf rescue board, also provides a rest station and can allow the teacher to maintain a clear view of the class.

Staying in pairs

In open-water environments it is wise to ensure that everyone has a 'buddy'. If there is a spare person, have one threesome. The teacher should not be used as a buddy.

SUN SAFETY

Most aquatic activities are outdoors and, consequently, in an environment where participants can be exposed to high levels of ultraviolet radiation. Exposure to the sun's ultraviolet rays is known to be one of the main causes of skin cancer. The most dangerous years are during childhood. Exposure to the sun during these years considerably increases the likelihood of skin cancer later in life.

Prevention is very important and the following measures are recommended to reduce the risk of skin cancer.

- Avoid the sun in the middle of the day (11 a.m. – 3 p.m. daylight saving time). Even when it is cool or cloudy the sun's radiation can still be damaging, so it is important to cover up even when it is not hot.
- Wear protective clothing such as a wide-brimmed hat and a long-sleeved shirt.
- Ensure a broad spectrum, water-resistant sunscreen (SPF 30+) is applied.
- Utilise the shade where possible (beach umbrellas, trees, shade structures).

Teachers should ensure that students and themselves are well protected during swimming and water safety programs.

It is essential that teachers encourage students to observe these safe practices when classes are conducted in the open.

When moving from an indoor to outdoor area, students should be given prior notice in order to properly prepare their sun safety procedures.

TEACHING TIP

Where possible, sunscreen should be applied by a parent or carer, but in situations where this is not possible, teachers have a duty of care to ensure that students are well protected from the sun.

At a river venue

At a river venue the teacher should remain on the down-current side of the group wherever possible. Grab ropes, placed across the current downstream from the working area, may be grasped in an emergency.

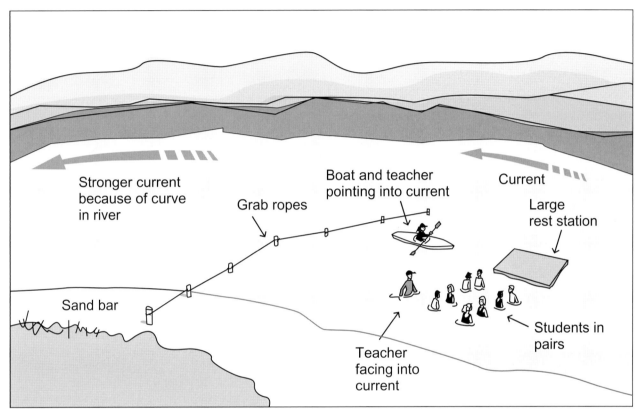

River venue

Extremes of temperature

Extremes of temperature, either heat or cold, can be dangerous to some people and are uncomfortable for all. Long periods in direct sun or cold winds should be avoided unless students are suitably dressed.

Thunderstorm

During thunderstorms and lightning there is a safety risk in participating in aquatic activities in outdoor venues. When lightning is within 10 km of the facility — that is, there is 30 seconds or less between a lightning strike and a thunderclap — all aquatic activities including swimming and water safety lessons should cease. The teacher of swimming and water safety should evacuate all their students from the water to a covered area (not trees, gazebos or marquees). Lessons may resume once the lightning has moved greater than 10 km away or, as a general rule, suspend activities until 30 minutes after the last thunderclap.

Teachers should always have planned some dry activities to be used when the students cannot participate in the water activities. Teachers should ensure the students and themselves are dry and warm before commencing activities.

Safety behaviour

Information about emergency procedures and dangerous places, conditions and behaviours (e.g. pushing in) should be provided, and its importance emphasised from the outset. Students should never dive or jump in the water at the beginning of a lesson, but rather sit down and slide in. Students must be encouraged to keep their heads above water and in clear sight when not practising a skill or drill.

The medical history

The medical history of all students should be known, particularly in regard to conditions that may affect participation in a swimming and water safety program, such as epilepsy, heart disease and asthma. Enrolment forms should include a section on medical history of the participants, including any parents/carers actively involved in the lesson. Teachers must be aware of their students' medical conditions to enable them to program lessons appropriately, ensure safety at all times and be ready to deal with any emergency.

Behaviour in emergencies

Emergency procedures should be practised even though it is hoped an emergency will never arise. Don't assume that emergencies will never happen to you!

The class

The class is the teacher's responsibility. In an emergency, teachers must not leave the class alone. If necessary, another teacher should take control of two classes temporarily, with the students out of the water.

Check the roll

The teacher should check the roll at the beginning and end of each lesson, and do 'head counts' during lessons, particularly when classes are large and conditions crowded.

PREPARING FOR AN EMERGENCY

All involved in swimming and water safety programs must know their roles in case of an emergency. This will ensure smooth and efficient responses and avoid indecision and replication of tasks.

Class safety and emergency procedures

The safety of students in a class must be the primary consideration of teachers at all times. In agreeing to teach students, whether in a paid or voluntary capacity, teachers are always responsible for the safety of the group. They are said to be '*in loco parentis*' (in place of the parent).

At some venues, additional safety support may be provided, such as qualified pool attendants or lifeguards. Irrespective of such support being available, ultimate responsibility for the safety of groups being taught falls on the AUSTSWIM teacher. It is therefore essential that teachers have developed an emergency plan and that they are well versed in safety procedures, rescue and after-care techniques.

The majority of swimming pool complexes have established, well-documented emergency procedures. Teachers using these venues must thoroughly familiarise themselves with the emergency procedures being practised at the venues they are using.

It is strongly recommended that each teacher develop a class emergency plan that complements existing emergency procedures.

Emergency procedures must be continually practised and reviewed.

Developing an emergency plan

Thorough preparation is essential to ensure the smooth and efficient mobilisation of an emergency plan.

Often emergency procedures look great on paper, but then flaws are discovered during an accident. Obviously, for any plan to operate efficiently, it must be practised regularly. Emergency drills will only operate effectively if all teachers at a venue, plus the staff and pool manager (if applicable), have discussed and become familiar with their respective roles. If the practice sessions do not work smoothly at first, further practice sessions will be necessary until they do. If the practices continue to be unsuccessful, an alternative plan must be considered. Emergency drills are important. They should not be seen as a break from lessons, a joke or a game.

Aquatic facility and program managers are generally responsible for establishing an emergency plan for their specific venue. Employees should have access to a copy of the emergency plan, be well versed in the procedures and experience a 'practice drill'. Teachers of swimming and water safety need to ensure they are familiar with the emergency plan and what their responsibilities are should an emergency occur.

Prior notice of the practising of emergency procedures should be provided to students, parents and carers. A simple note advising that 'emergency procedures will be practised at this venue during the next 3 weeks' (for example) is quite adequate. This will ensure effective communication with all and allow time for appropriate discussion and preparation.

The development of a checklist will indicate if the facility has the appropriate equipment for an emergency. The following points must be considered in developing a checklist:

EMERGENCY CHECKLIST

- ❏ Location of nearest telephone.
  - ❏ Is it always accessible?
- ❏ Location and telephone number of nearest ambulance.
- ❏ Location and telephone number of nearest medical assistance (if ambulance is not readily available).
- ❏ Means of transport to medical assistance.
- ❏ Location of first-aid kit.
  - ❏ Is it always accessible?
  - ❏ Is it always unlocked?
  - ❏ Is it well stocked?
- ❏ Location of rescue equipment (e.g. ropes, poles, rescue tubes, kickboards).
- ❏ Names of trained first-aid and lifesaving personnel on site.
- ❏ Emergency signal to be used:
  - ❏ bell
  - ❏ whistle (including the number of times sound is heard, e.g. one long whistle)
  - ❏ siren.
- ❏ Statement of emergency procedures to be implemented:
  - ❏ emergency action
  - ❏ role of staff involved
  - ❏ after-care actions.
- ❏ Supplementary list of other helpful agencies (e.g. St John Ambulance Australia, Fire Brigade, SES, Poisons Information Bureau).

It is disturbing in an emergency situation to discover that the telephone is locked away during lunchtime and nobody knows where to find the key, or that the cupboard has been tidied and the first-aid box has been removed. Access to emergency equipment,

particularly a telephone with a direct line, must be maintained at all times.

AUSTSWIM teachers working in natural water environments have to be particularly well prepared for emergency situations. Communication and immediate access to assistance have to be carefully and thoroughly considered and an emergency plan needs to be specifically developed for the working area.

In determining emergency procedures, teachers must consider the minimum number of competent people required, should an emergency situation arise. Consideration should be given as to who:

- leaves to get assistance
- looks after the class/es
- performs the 'rescue' (if necessary).

The figure on page 190 is an example of the actions that might be planned for three people.

Everyone involved in an aquatic program must know their role should an emergency situation arise. This will ensure the smooth and efficient implementation of their emergency actions and avoid indecision and replication of tasks.

After an emergency

Teachers must be familiar with the actions required by their class organisers or employers immediately following an accident. This might involve providing information to the:

- pool manager
- local council
- school principal
- regional office
- education department.

In all cases a detailed written accident report needs to be completed and signed by competent witnesses (particularly those directly involved). Details of times and actions taken are very important. Remember that legal action often takes years to come to court. It will be very difficult for teachers to recall exactly what occurred years before!

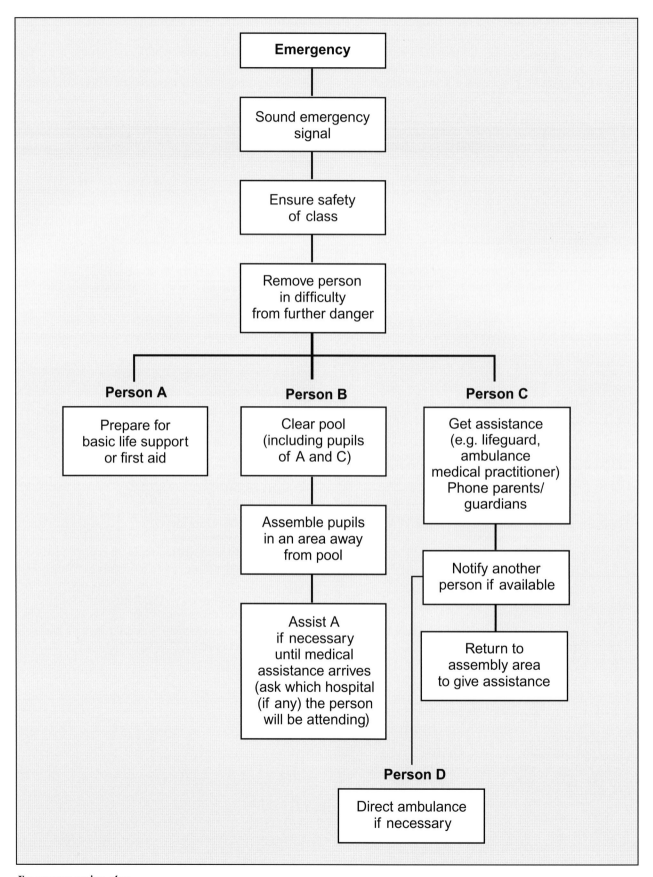

Emergency action plan

REVIEW QUESTIONS

1 What should the structure of a lesson comprise of?
2 Explain the pros and cons of a teacher being in or out of the water when teaching a class.
3 What are the factors a teacher needs to consider when reviewing a lesson?
4 Where can full details of the recommended AUSTSWIM student–teacher ratios be found?
5 Describe the advantages and disadvantages of using teaching equipment.
   List as many types of equipment that you can think of.
6 What are the 'safety' considerations when conducting an aquatic program in open water?
   Describe what should be included on an emergency checklist.

Appendices

AUSTSWIM Teacher
Code of Behaviour

APPENDIX 1

AUSTSWIM TEACHER CODE OF BEHAVIOUR

The primary objective of the AUSTSWIM Teacher Code of Behaviour is to ensure AUSTSWIM teachers provide safe swimming and water safety programs at all times and that a high level of instruction is delivered. The AUSTSWIM Teacher Code of Behaviour will:

- encourage public confidence in aquatic education
- publicise AUSTSWIM's expectations of AUSTSWIM teachers
- demonstrate that AUSTSWIM teachers accept a standard of practice
- provide a benchmark for appropriate aquatic behaviour.

All trainees for and holders of AUSTSWIM qualifications agree to:

- Abide by the AUSTSWIM Teacher Code of Behaviour, qualification regulations and policies, including:
  - maintaining AUSTSWIM qualifications
  - participating in regular professional development opportunities.
- Follow policy for enforcement of this code:
  - referring to established procedures for appealing against assessment results
  - accepting any judgments made by AUSTSWIM and/or its agents
  - teaching within the limits of competence deemed by the AUSTSWIM qualifications held.
- Follow AUSTSWIM policy and guidelines relating to safety, class ratios, emergency procedures and duty of care.
- Follow relevant legislation regarding working with children. Relevant state and territory laws are available at: www.ausport.gov.au/ethics/legischild.asp.
- Promote the participation of all Australians in safe and enjoyable swimming and water safety programs conducted by qualified personnel. Teachers will:
  - promote and deliver only safe and enjoyable aquatic activities
  - show respect for the health, safety and welfare of participants and colleagues.
- Enhance water safety knowledge while developing swimming, water safety and survival skills, by:
  - providing a balanced program of swimming and water safety
  - providing a planned and sequential program of aquatic skill development based on the needs of each participant.
- Provide equal opportunity for all to learn swimming, water safety and survival skills, by:
  - modifying the program to cater for those with disabilities, injuries, special learning needs, cultural needs, adult learners and personal readiness.
- Ensure that all persons under tuition are treated with the courtesy and respect deserving of all people, irrespective of individual differences and needs, by:
  - refraining from any discriminatory practices by treating everyone equally
  - being alert and respond to any form of abuse between participants.
- Represent AUSTSWIM and the swimming and water safety teaching industry in a professional manner without bringing the teaching profession or AUSTSWIM into disrepute, by:
  - being a role model for other AUSTSWIM teachers
  - behaving professionally and accepting responsibility for your actions
  - extending professional courtesy to other AUSTSWIM teachers, industry colleagues, participants and parents
  - refraining from any form of verbal, physical or emotional abuse
  - refraining from any form of sexual harassment towards participants
  - refraining from using the influence of a teaching position to encourage inappropriate intimacy between teacher and participants
  - ensuring physical support is only provided to facilitate learning or safe performance
  - ensuring all personal and sensitive information collected be treated confidentially and in accordance with privacy laws.

In addition to the obligations set out above, comply, in all circumstances, with relevant state, territory and national laws including, but not limited to, the areas of equal opportunity, anti-discrimination, child protection, privacy, criminal history checks, and occupational health and safety. If you are unsure about any of your obligations, you should contact AUSTSWIM and seek assistance.

POLICY FOR BREACH OF AUSTSWIM TEACHER CODE OF BEHAVIOUR

AUSTSWIM, on receiving a complaint for a breach of behaviour, will form a review panel to investigate issues relating to AUSTSWIM candidates', teachers' and course presenters' compliance with the AUSTSWIM Teacher Code of Behaviour.

The review panel will investigate and review the complaint and make a recommendation for action to AUSTSWIM.

If a teacher is found in breach of the code the review panel may, depending on the nature of the breach, recommend a reprimand, suspension for a period of time or deregistration as an AUSTSWIM teacher.

Learn to Swim and Water Safety enrolment form (sample)

APPENDIX 2

LEARN TO SWIM AND WATER SAFETY ENROLMENT FORM (SAMPLE)

This consent form is provided as an example of the type of information that may be collected when enrolling students in swimming and water safety programs.

Student's details

	Student name	Sex	Date of birth	Please list any health issues that may affect your child's participation in lessons (e.g. asthma)
1				

Parent/guardian details

Full name of parent/guardian:		
Postal address:		
Contact number (H):	(M):	(W):
Sex M/F:	Email:	

Emergency contact details

In case of an emergency we require contact details of a person other than the person who will be attending the lessons with the child/children.

Full name:		
Relationship to 1. child:	2. carer:	
Contact number (H):	(M):	(W):

Parent/carer details (for parent/carer and child classes)

This information is required of the parent/carer who will be participating in programs where the parent/carer must be in the water (e.g. infant classes).

Parent/ carer name	Sex	Please list any health issues that may affect your participation in your child's lessons (e.g. asthma)

Terms and conditions

Medical release and declaration

I authorise the teachers to obtain medical assistance which they deem necessary should an accident occur, and agree to pay all medical expenses incurred on behalf of the above student and carer. I submit the attached medical information about my child and include other relevant information and details of limitations which he/she has for the activity concerned. I further authorise qualified practitioners to administer anaesthetic if such an eventuality arises.

Privacy policy

I understand that the information I have provided is collected and held in accordance with the provisions of the Privacy Act. I understand that the information I have provided is necessary for the service to be provided. I acknowledge and agree that the information will only be used to facilitate the service and to advise me of matters relating to the service. I understand that I will be able to access and alter information that has been supplied. I acknowledge that if I do not wish to receive promotional material I must advise in writing.

Parent/Carer Signature: ……………………………………………………… Date: ………… / ………… / …………

Accident report form (sample)

ACCIDENT REPORT FORM (SAMPLE)

The following information must be gathered and recorded immediately after an accident/incident by the teacher or designated person. At the majority of venues it will be the lifeguards' responsibility to record these details, however teachers may need to assist with information.

Accident report form

In the event of an accident, please complete and forward to employer immediately.	
A. Details of injured person	
A.1 Name:	
A.2 Address:	
A.3 Telephone number:	
A.4 Age (at time of accident, in years):	A.5 Date of birth:
B. Witnesses	
B.1 Name of teacher on duty:	
B.2 Details of witnesses:	
B.3 Home address:	
B.4 Telephone:	
C. Details of accident	
C.1 Date:	C.2 Time (a.m./p.m.)
C.3 Place (details):	
C.4 Description:	
C.5 Nature of injury:	
C.6 Cause of accident:	
D. Action taken (first aid, parents contacted, ambulance called, reported only, etc.):	
E. Other comments:	
F. Details and signature of person filling out form:	
Name (please print):	Signature:
Date:	Venue:	Program:

Medical considerations

Asthma

CONDITION

- A breathing problem resulting from sudden or progressive narrowing of the airways.
- Causes may be physical, chemical or psychological, including allergies, infection and exercise.

SIGNS/SYMPTOMS

- Desire to sit up. Often starts with cough or chest tightness.
- Often worse at night or with exercise.
- Moderate to severe breathing difficulty.
- Wheezing is a later development and may indicate 50% or more lung capacity reduction.
- Sweating and pallor.
- Quiet and subdued manner.
- Possible loss of consciousness.

MANAGEMENT

- Danger–response–airway–breathing–circulation (DRABC).
- Sit the person upright.
- Encourage quiet gentle nasal breathing.
- Give reassurance and advise the person to stay calm.
- Ensure that there is access to fresh air.
- Check for personal medication and help administer as required.
- If the person is not settling, or visibly improving, get him/her to hospital as soon as possible. Asthma can be a life-threatening condition.

Common cold/influenza

CONDITION

- Caused by many different types and strains of virus.
- There is danger not just from the cold virus, but also from secondary bacterial infections.

SIGNS/SYMPTOMS

- Fever (fever and raised resting heart rate are usually an indicator of a more serious infection).
- Sneezing.
- Sniffing.
- Cough (may be an indication of asthma or bronchitis).
- Blocked nose (can lead to Eustachian tube dysfunction and possible middle ear infections).
- Sore throat.
- Earache.

MANAGEMENT

- Rest and drink plenty of fluid. Consider the following:
  - never train when sick as this can lead to more serious conditions such as chronic fatigue or even injuries
  - advise not to swim in confined areas such as pools, both in the patient's interests and in those of other swimmers.
- Seek medical assistance if symptoms persist.

Cramp

CONDITIONS

Thought to be related to an inadequate flow of blood to local muscle during periods of peak demand. May be related to dehydration, inadequate carbohydrate load, or neural back problems.

SIGNS/SYMPTOMS

A sudden, painful involuntary spasm of muscle.

MANAGEMENT

- Help the student to leave the water.
- Warm and stretch the muscle.
- Address possible causes or refer to a doctor if it becomes a chronic problem.

Diabetes

CONDITION

- Failure of the body to produce sufficient insulin to assist in the clearing of sugar from the bloodstream into muscle cells.
- Two types of problem:
  1. insulin-dependent diabetes (needing to be treated with insulin)
  2. mature-onset (usually) non-insulin-dependent diabetes (may respond to diet, weight loss, or oral medications).

SIGNS/SYMPTOMS

- Hyperglycaemia (very high blood sugar levels):
  - extreme thirst
  - frequent toilet visits (urination)
  - fast pulse rate
  - drowsiness
  - hot, dry skin
  - glucose in urine
  - severe cases can lead to vomiting, stomach aches, and laboured breathing from ketoacidosis
  - may lead to coma.
- Hypoglycaemia (low blood sugar levels):
  - dizziness, weakness and trembling
  - hunger
  - fast pulse rate
  - pallor
  - sweating and some numbness (fingertips)
  - confusion if severe
  - can lead to loss of consciousness.

MANAGEMENT OF HIGH BLOOD SUGAR

- If unconscious: danger–response–airway–breathing–circulation (DRABC) — seek medical help immediately.
- If conscious, give sugar-free drinks.
- Help the person to administer insulin.
- Seek medical aid.

MANAGEMENT OF LOW BLOOD SUGAR

- If unconscious: danger–response–airway–breathing–circulation (DRABC) — seek medical help immediately.
- If conscious, give sugar, glucose or a sweet drink liberally every 15 minutes.
- Ask student/parent/carer for information if possible.
- Look for medical alert bracelet or warning cards.
- Loosen tight clothing and make comfortable.

Ear — middle-ear infection

CONDITION

Infection of the middle ear usually due to insufficient drainage through a blocked Eustachian tube. This can lead to perforation of the eardrum and a discharge. At this point the pain mostly disappears.

SIGNS/SYMPTOMS

- Persistent earache.
- Fever.
- Mild to severe deafness.
- Ear discharge.

MANAGEMENT

Seek immediate medical attention.

Ear — simple earache

CONDITION

Typically comes with exposure to the cold and will disappear as soon as the swimmer leaves the water and warms up.

SIGNS/SYMPTOMS

Earache.

MANAGEMENT

If no relief after a short time, suspect middle-ear infection (see above) and consult a doctor.

Ear — tropical ear

CONDITION

- Infection of the skin in the canal of the outer ear that can affect:
  - all the skin of the ear canal
  - the root of the hair follicle, causing a boil to form.

Requires lengthy treatment to avoid frequent recurrence. Occurs in tropical regions. May be caused by inadequate drying of the ear canal after swimming.

SIGNS/SYMPTOMS

- Itchy ears.
- Pain.
- Hearing loss.
- Discharge.

MANAGEMENT

- Seek medical advice.
- Use ear drops to settle infections.
- Clear the ear of dead skin (medically qualified person required).
- Possibly get fitted ear plugs.

Epilepsy

CONDITION

- Brief disturbance of the electrical activity of the brain.
- Seizures occurring at variable intervals. Can be *grand mal* (generalised seizures) 51% or *petit mal* (staring spells) 8% or both (41%).
- Most common in the age groups 0–2 years, 4–8 years and around puberty.

SIGNS/SYMPTOMS

- Sudden loss of consciousness.
- Loss of muscle tone.
- Stiffening of the body and clenching of teeth.
- Rolling eyes and foaming at the mouth.
- Spasm of the larynx and sometimes loss of bladder or rectal control.
- On regaining consciousness, possibly confusion and no awareness of what happened.

MANAGEMENT

- Danger–response–airway–breathing–circulation (DRABC).
- Protect from injury; do not restrict movements.
- Do not put anything in the mouth.
- Place casualty on their side as soon as possible when seizure is over.
- Make warm and comfortable.
- Allow casualty to sleep; check airway, breathing, circulation.
- Seek medical aid if seizure continues for more than 10 minutes.

Eye irritation

CONDITION

Sometimes caused by impure water, such as water that is salty or chemically imbalanced.

SIGNS/SYMPTOMS

- Sore eyes.
- Red eyes.
- Constant rubbing and/or blinking.

MANAGEMENT

- Use eye drops such as Visine.
- If persistent, advise use of goggles.
- Be aware of the possibility of conjunctivitis, which may require antibiotic drops.

Heart attack

CONDITION

Many different causes, such as physical or mental stress, or associated diseases.

SIGNS/SYMPTOMS

- Pain or discomfort in the centre of the chest lasting for more than 10 minutes.
- Pain (usually like pressure or tightness) spreading to the shoulder, arm, throat or jaw.
- Anxiety, confusion or distress.
- Shortness of breath.
- Irregular pulse.
- Collapse, leading to absence of pulse.
- Pale, cold, clammy skin.

MANAGEMENT

- If unconscious:
  - danger–response–airway–breathing–circulation (DRABC) — seek medical help
  - turn the person on to the side.
- If conscious:
  - seek medical aid quickly
  - sit the person up and quietly try to reassure him/her
  - in case of dizziness, lie down and turn the person on to their side.

Plantar warts (papilloma)

CONDITION

Frequently occurring on the sole of the foot among swimmers. Caused by highly contagious virus and easily spread in swimming pools or showers.

SIGNS/SYMPTOMS

- Appearing singly or in groups as small blackheads.
- Pain when walking.

MANAGEMENT

- Seek medical/podiatry help.
- Possibly exclude person from swimming program until medical clearance is received or at least wear thongs in the showers.

Sunburn and windburn

CONDITION

Inflammation of the skin caused by exposure to sun or wind.

SIGNS/SYMPTOMS

- Red, swollen and possibly blistered skin.
- Pain in the affected areas.

MANAGEMENT

- Advise cold showers.
- Can use oral analgesic (e.g. Codalgin or Panadeine) for pain control in adults.
- Liquid Panadol or Nurofen may be helpful for children.
- Apply cool, moist compresses to the burnt area.
- Rest in cool place.
- For young babies, or others with blistered skin, seek medical attention.

PREVENTION

- Encourage protection against excessive exposure (children are particularly susceptible).
- Ensure protective clothing is worn including suitable protective swimwear when in the water.

Tinea (athlete's foot)

CONDITION

Fungal infection usually between toes or can appear as jock rash in groin.

SIGNS/SYMPTOMS

- Often goes unnoticed but can be seen as wetness and peeling, macerated skin between the toes, most often starting between the fourth and fifth toes.
- If neglected can invade the nail beds, leading to thickened, hard, unattractive nails.

MANAGEMENT

- Anti-fungal cream is to be rubbed in very well between the toes twice daily, and continued for at least a week after the skin has fully healed.
- Avoid wearing woollen socks and try to air feet whenever possible.
- Always dry between the toes and dry the groin very well after swimming.

PREVENTION

Remember prevention is better than cure so dry your toes and perhaps wear thongs in the showers.

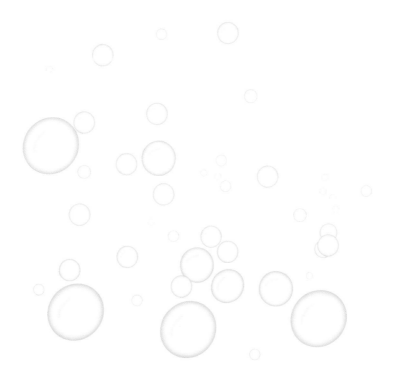

Medical considerations and criteria for exclusion of students who are unwell

A medical form detailing any special conditions should be completed prior to the commencement of classes, and aquatics teachers should be familiar with students in their class who have special needs. Where parents participate in the program a medical form should also be completed by them to indicate their own health status (see Appendix 2 for sample).

Exclusion of a student from an aquatic program is recommended when there is a health risk to other participants. While there are no specific recommendations for exclusion of participants from public swimming pools or aquatic programs, the normal guidelines for exclusion from group settings, such as school programs, are applicable.

Parents should be encouraged to avoid bringing students to class when they have a fever or other symptoms such as a rash or runny nose. These symptoms are often the signs of infection and the affected students are a risk to other students in the class. Students who have any symptoms of diarrhoea or vomiting should be excluded until they are fully recovered. Students who are unwell will also be at greater risk of hypothermia and will not be able to attend to and gain full benefit from the program. Parents should be helped to understand that students will only benefit from the program when they are healthy and able to actively participate in and enjoy the program.

GUIDELINES FOR EXCLUSION

The following guidelines are from *Staying Healthy in Child Care — Preventing infectious diseases in child care*, 4th edition, published by the National Health and Medical Research Council (NHMRC), Australian Government (December 2006).

Disease or condition	Exclusion of cases	Exclusion of contacts
Chickenpox	Exclude until all blisters have dried. This is usually at least 5 days after the rash first appeared in unimmunised children and less in immunised children.	Any child with an immune deficiency (e.g. leukaemia) or receiving chemotherapy should be excluded for their own protection. Otherwise, not excluded.
Conjunctivitis (acute infectious)	Exclude until the discharge from the eyes has stopped unless doctor has diagnosed a non-infectious conjunctivitis.	Not excluded.
Diarrhoea (no organism identified)	Exclude until there has not been a loose bowel motion for 24 hours.	Not excluded.
Diphtheria	Exclude until medical certificate of recovery is received following at least two negative throat swabs, the first swab not less than 24 hours after finishing a course of antibiotics followed by another swab 48 hours later.	Exclude contacts that live in the same house until cleared to return by an appropriate health authority.
Giardiasis (diarrhoea)	Exclude until there has not been a loose bowel motion for 24 hours.	Not excluded.
Head lice (pediculosis)	Exclusion is NOT necessary if effective treatment is commenced prior to the next day at child care (i.e. the child doesn't need to be sent home immediately if head lice are detected).	Not excluded.
Hepatitis A	Exclude until a medical certificate of recovery is received, but not before 7 days after the onset of jaundice.	Not excluded.
Hepatitis B	Exclusion is NOT necessary.	Not excluded.

Disease or condition	Exclusion of cases	Exclusion of contacts
Impetigo (school sores)	Exclude until appropriate antibiotic treatment has commenced. Any sores on exposed skin should be covered with a watertight dressing.	Not excluded.
Leprosy	Exclude until approval to return has been given by an appropriate health authority.	Not excluded.
Measles	Exclude for 4 days after the onset of the rash.	Immunised and immune contacts are not excluded. Non-immunised contacts of a case are to be excluded from child care until 14 days after the first day of appearance of rash in the last case, unless immunised within 72 hours of first contact during the infectious period with the first case. All immuno-compromised children should be excluded until 14 days after the first day of appearance of rash in the last case.
Meningococcal infection	Exclude until appropriate antibiotic treatment has been completed.	Not excluded.
Mumps	Exclude for 9 days after onset of swelling.	Not excluded.
Ringworm/tinea	Exclude until the day after appropriate antifungal treatment has commenced.	Not excluded.
Rotavirus infection	Children are to be excluded from the centre until there has not been a loose bowel motion or vomiting for 24 hours.	Not excluded.
Rubella (German measles)	Exclude until fully recovered or for at least 4 days after the onset of the rash.	Not excluded.
Scabies	Exclude until the day after appropriate treatment has commenced.	Not excluded.
Shigella infection	Exclude until there has not been a loose bowel motion for 24 hours.	Not excluded.
Streptococcal sore throat (including scarlet fever)	Exclude until the person has received antibiotic treatment for at least 24 hours and feels well.	Not excluded.
Tuberculosis (TB)	Exclude until medical certificate is produced from an appropriate health authority.	Not excluded.
Typhoid, paratyphoid	Exclude until medical certificate is produced from an appropriate health authority.	Not excluded unless a medical officer considers exclusion to be necessary.
Whooping cough (pertussis)	Exclude until 5 days after starting appropriate antibiotic treatment or for 21 days from the onset of coughing.	Contacts that live in the same house as the case and have received less than three doses of pertussis vaccine are to be excluded from the centre until they have had 5 days of an appropriate course of antibiotics. If antibiotics have not been taken, these contacts must be excluded for 21 days after their last exposure to the case while the person was infectious.

Games and activities

APPENDIX 6

GAMES AND ACTIVITIES

Following are some games and activities that teachers may use.

 Chain Reaction

NUMBER

Four or more.

ORGANISATION

In a circle.

AREA

Shallow water.

EQUIPMENT

None.

Description

In waist-deep water, the group stands in a circle. The teacher chooses the starter, who must then do an action (e.g. blow bubbles) and each student in turn must copy. The next turn goes to the student on the right of the starter. It is then their turn to pick an activity, adding to the previous one.

 City Bridges

NUMBER

Up to whole class.

ORGANISATION

Small groups or teams of about four, well spaced.

AREA

Knee-deep to waist-deep water.

EQUIPMENT

None.

Description

Two members of each group join hands and form an arch. The remainder of the group stand one behind the other, each holding onto the waist of the person in front and ready to pass under the arch. On the word 'go' each group, as a 'train', passes first under its own arch and then under every other arch. The first team to pass under all the arches and back through its own is the winner.

Dodgem Cars

NUMBER

Equal teams.

ORGANISATION

- Fit noodle around base of spine, straddle legs over either end of the noodle.
- Form two parallel lines (facing one another) across wide pool area.

AREA

Waist-deep to deeper water (ensure all students are comfortable and capable in deep water).

EQUIPMENT

One water noodle per person.

Description

The objective is to enhance body orientation and balance skills, it will improve endurance and strength with forward and back sculling.

- At command of 'go' students scull towards one another. Attempt to grab opposition by the feet and 'flip' them backwards.
- Once 'flipped', a student is out of the game. Continue until there is one person left.
- Students who are 'flipped' and out of the game form an outer circle and, while still 'sitting' on their noodles, create turbulence for the students still remaining in the game.

Flashcards

NUMBER

Four or more.

ORGANISATION

In a line facing the teacher.

AREA

Shallow water.

EQUIPMENT

Flashcards, e.g. $(2 + \ldots = 4)$ or $(5 - \ldots = 3)$.

Description

Students must collect from the surface, or bottom, rings or ping-pong balls that would total the numbers missing from the cards.

Flutter-Ring Drop

NUMBER

Groups of up to six.

ORGANISATION

With individuals or small groups.

AREA

Waist-deep water.

EQUIPMENT

A set of flutter rings.

Description

The teacher 'throws' in the flutter rings, which slowly descend. The teacher can nominate the number or colour of the ring each student must retrieve.

Follow the Leader

NUMBER

Four or more.

ORGANISATION

Students line up behind the leader.

AREA

Shallow water.

EQUIPMENT

None or hoops, dive rings, etc.

Description

In waist-deep water, students line up behind the 'leader' who takes them through a number of movements that the teacher asks of them (e.g. walking, running, forwards and backwards, zigzagging, hopping, picking up a ring, swimming through a hoop, and so forth). Change leaders to give all a go.

Giant Glide

NUMBER

Up to 10.

ORGANISATION

Students line up approximately 1.5–2.0 m apart.

AREA

Shallow to waist-deep water — minimum of 10 m length is required for maximum benefit. For safety make sure students don't get pushed into a wall!

EQUIPMENT

None required.

Description

The objective of this game is for the students to experience gliding and the exhilaration of gliding fast!

- The first student pushes off the end of the wall face down in a streamlined body position.
- When they reach the second student, they are further propelled in the same direction by a forceful push to hips or feet.
- This continues until the student needs to take a breath or reaches the end of the line.
- Students rotate positions so all experience the glide.
- This activity can also be done on the back.

Huff 'n' Puff

NUMBER

Small group to whole class.

ORGANISATION

Individual players, each using a unit of equipment, or a team relay race.

AREA

Waist-deep water.

EQUIPMENT

Ping-pong ball.

Description

The players stand side by side at the starting point, each with a ping-pong ball. On the command 'go' they enter the water and float the ball, then blow it along the surface of the water to the finish line. The ball may only be touched at the start and the finish.

Kickboard Scramble

NUMBER

Up to 10.

ORGANISATION

Split students into two even teams.

AREA

Shallow water (clearly defined area).

EQUIPMENT

Kickboards (can be replaced by other equipment, e.g. balls, toys and so forth).

Description

The objective of this game is to develop confidence in shallow water.

- Each group starts at opposite sides of the teaching area.
- In the centre place an uneven number of kickboards (or other equipment).
- On teacher's signal, all students race to collect one board each which they take back to their base.
- Winning team will have at least one more board than the other.

Kickboard Toss

NUMBER

Small group to whole class.

ORGANISATION

Team of four working from edge to hoop and back; hoop 10 metres from edge (or at distance appropriate to ability of players).

AREAS

Shallow water.

EQUIPMENT

A tethered hoop and three kickboards for each team.

Description

Members of each team line up on the edge of the pool opposite a hoop. The aim is to throw the kickboards so that they land within the hoop; each player uses all three kickboards and scores one point for each successful throw. When number 1 has thrown each board, that player enters the water, retrieves the boards and returns them to number 2, and so on until all team members have had a turn. The team with the highest score wins.

Noodle Sculling

NUMBER

Small group to whole class.

ORGANISATION

Fit noodle around base of spine, straddle legs over either end of the noodle.

AREA

Waist-deep to deeper water (ensure all students are comfortable and capable in deep water).

EQUIPMENT

One water noodle per person.

Description

The objective is to enhance body orientation and balance skills, it will improve endurance and strength with forward and back sculling.

- Students maintain balance in upright 'sitting' position.
- Practice sculling to target (forward sculling) and back to start (back sculling).
- Practice lying back and recovering to stable 'sitting' position.

Shipwreck

NUMBER

Up to 10.

ORGANISATION

Students are placed in a clearly defined area.

AREA

Shallow water for beginners — can be done in deeper water for advanced students.

EQUIPMENT

None.

Description

The objective of this game is to be able to effectively climb out of the pool.

The students respond to the teacher's commands:

- 'Scrub the deck' — force the water surface into waves.
- 'Captain's coming' — all students salute.
- 'SHARK' — all students must climb completely out of the water.

Sky Board

NUMBER

Up to 10.

ORGANISATION

Students line up approximately 1 m apart. They should be encouraged to blow out through their nose when submerging to ensure water doesn't go up it!

AREA

Waist-deep to deeper water.

EQUIPMENT

One kickboard per group — can be substituted for a ball.

Description

The objective of this game is to develop floating and balancing skills.

- While sculling on their back, the first student in each team gathers the kickboard in their feet.
- They then pass the kickboard over their head and pass it to the next member of their team.
- This continues until all team members have a turn.

Splish Splash

NUMBER

Six or more.

ORGANISATION

In two teams.

AREA

Shallow to waist-deep water.

EQUIPMENT

One large plastic jug and one kickboard per team.

Description

In waist-deep water each team forms a circle. A plastic jug with no lid is placed in the centre on a kickboard. On the signal 'go', all students begin splashing water into their team's jug. No student may touch the jug. The team to fill the jug first is the winner.

Weed Wall

NUMBER

Small group to whole class.

ORGANISATION

Team of four to six.

AREA

Shallow water.

EQUIPMENT

Strips of plastic attached to weighted hoops (use garbage bags).

Description

Teams line up at the edge of the pool in a crocodile line with the 'wall of weeds' in place along the middle of the playing area. Players in turn enter the water, wade across the pool through the weeds, touch the other side and wade back through the weeds to the starting point. The first team to finish is the winner.

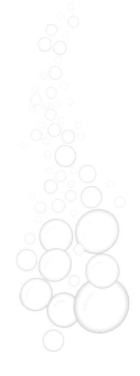

Learning characteristics of different age groups

APPENDIX 7

LEARNING CHARACTERISTICS OF DIFFERENT AGE GROUPS

Teachers need to work in with the development level of the class. A brief outline of the various age characteristics is given below and each age group is discussed, along with some implications for teaching that group.

> It should be understood that the age groupings are only generalisations. As in all teaching, it is unwise to assume that the generalisation covers all individuals.

THE PRESCHOOL CHILD (4–6 YEARS AGE GROUP)

Age group characteristics

- Relatively close to their babyhood experiences.
- Rapid growth slows down to steady increase by age of six.
- Heart and lungs are small in proportion to height and weight.
- Outstandingly active.
- Slow coordination development.
- Child egocentric — first experience in a homogeneous group.
- Curious and creative.
- Attention span is very short — love repetition.
- Child unable to focus quickly or accurately.
- Limited vocabulary and few fears.

Implications/meeting needs

- 'Big muscle' activities followed by rest periods.
- Teach skills of body control.
- Repeat activities often.
- Encourage cooperative group activity.
- Simple directions.
- Water needs to be shallow to enable the children to stand comfortably.
- Creativity stimulated by bright colours — use colourful balls, hoops, blocks, dive rings, kickboards.
- Avoid formal instructions — emphasis mostly on safe water experiences.
- Be patient and accept small gains.
- Generate the fun element and maintain interest.
- Rhymes and rhythms can be of great value.

THE EARLY PRIMARY SCHOOL CHILD (6–8 YEARS AGE GROUP)

Age group characteristics

- Rate of structural growth moderate and steady — craving for exercise.
- Health precarious — low resistance, poor endurance.
- Coordination improving.
- Intensely individualistic — desires adult approval.
- Attention span short and retention poor.
- Reactions slow.
- Eye focus not fully developed.
- Sex differences are not of great consequence.

Implications/meeting needs

- 'Big muscle' activities provide most interest and value. Postural habits important — skeleton in formative stages.
- Vigorous activity for muscular development and endurance — rest and relaxation periods.
- Emphasise specific skills practice.
- Guidance in recognising the rights of others — leadership and group work.
- Responsibility — recognition for work well done.
- Repetition — simple directions and a few rules.
- Develop individuals by use of activities that reward success.
- Boys and girls have approximately same abilities and interests and should play together.

MIDDLE TO LATE PRIMARY SCHOOL CHILD (9–12 YEARS AGE GROUP)

Age group characteristics

- Height and weight steadily increase.
- Heart and lungs practically up to adult proportions.
- Health excellent, resistance and endurance improved.
- Muscular strength lags.
- Coordination and attention span improves. Interested in skill technique.
- Gregarious instincts develop. Group approval important.
- The gender differences are marked. Boys develop greater muscle power. Gender interests vary.

Implications/meeting needs

- Activities of sustained length — specific skills practiced in groups.
- Vigorous activities and the fun element can be maintained by using more organised games.
- Use of equipment can be exploited because of greater coordination.
- Beginners are really influenced by peer group.
- Onset of puberty is an awkward time and the widest range of skeletal maturity exists. Emotional instability is also apparent.
- More complicated water games and challenging activities can be systematically planned to advance coordination.

THE TEENAGER

Age group characteristics

- Usually personal reasons for not being able to swim.
- Very self-conscious.
- Reluctant to participate.
- Find excuses for not performing.
- Tension might cause their body actions to be stiff and awkward.

Implications/meeting needs

- Be considerate about circumstances and influences which have caused their lack of swimming ability; for example:
  - lack of opportunity
  - illness
  - physical disability
  - fear of performing in front of peers
  - past accident, causing fear of water and withdrawal.
- Need to overcome deep-seated fears.
- Need to give them rapid achievement.
- Provide a climate of learning which overcomes their fears and embarrassment.

THE ADULT

Age group characteristics

- Do not acquire new skills quite as easily as when younger.
- Physical abilities such as flexibility are reduced.
- Men find it more difficult to float than women.
- Embarrassment, misconceptions and pre-conceived fears can create tension and slow progress.
- Usually have a strong desire to persevere.

Implications/meeting needs

- Use similar techniques to those of teenage swimmers.
- May need to use flippers (fins) to help ankle flexibility.
- Help ease their tension and be aware of their embarrassment.
- Build on their motivation and desire to do well.

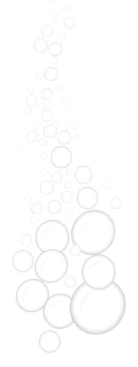

INDEX